# GENE TRANSFER, GENOME EDITING
## AND
# GENE THERAPY

Principles and Strategies

# GENE TRANSFER, GENOME EDITING
AND
# GENE THERAPY

## Principles and Strategies

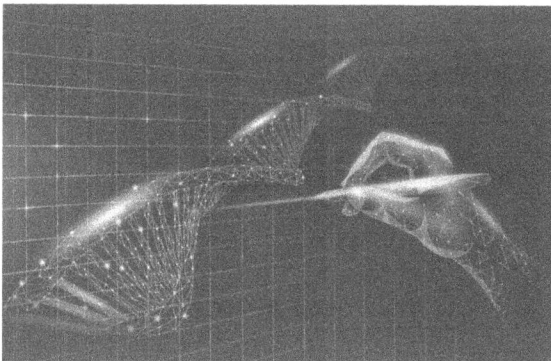

## Daniel Scherman
CNRS National Scientific Research Center, France

**World Scientific**

NEW JERSEY · LONDON · SINGAPORE · BEIJING · SHANGHAI · HONG KONG · TAIPEI · CHENNAI · TOKYO

*Published by*

World Scientific Publishing Europe Ltd.

57 Shelton Street, Covent Garden, London WC2H 9HE

*Head office:* 5 Toh Tuck Link, Singapore 596224

*USA office:* 27 Warren Street, Suite 401-402, Hackensack, NJ 07601

**Library of Congress Cataloging-in-Publication Data**

Names: Scherman, Daniel author
Title: Gene transfer, genome editing and gene therapy : principles and strategies / Daniel Scherman.
Description: London ; Hackensack, NJ : World Scientific Publishing Europe Ltd, [2026] |
  Includes bibliographical references and index. |
  Contents: Basic Definitions and General Principles -- Recombinant Viral Vectors:
  General Considerations -- Episomal Non-Integrative Viral Vectors:
  Adenovirus, AAV, and HSV-1 -- Integrative Vectors -- Non-Viral Gene
  Expression Vectors Derived from Retroviruses and Lentiviruses --
  Chemical Delivery of Non-Viral Vectors -- Physical Delivery of Non-Viral Vectors --
  CAR-T Cell Adoptive Immunotherapy -- Gene, Base, and Prime Editing --
  Antisense Deoxynucleotides (ASO) -- RNA Silencing and Small Interfering RNA --
  Challenges and Perspectives of ASO and siRNA Drugs.
Identifiers: LCCN 2025010553 | ISBN 9781800617520 hardcover |
  ISBN 9781800617537 ebook for institutions | ISBN 9781800617544 ebook for individuals
Subjects: MESH: Gene Transfer Techniques | Gene Editing | Genetic Therapy
Classification: LCC RB155.8 .S24 2026 | NLM QU 550
LC record available at https://lccn.loc.gov/2025010553

**British Library Cataloguing-in-Publication Data**
A catalogue record for this book is available from the British Library.

For any available supplementary material, please visit
https://www.worldscientific.com/worldscibooks/10.1142/Q0516#t=suppl

Desk Editors: Murali Appadurai/Cian Sacker Ooi

Typeset by Stallion Press
Email: enquiries@stallionpress.com

*This textbook is dedicated to the generous and enthusiastic scientists who opened my eyes to the beauty of gene-based therapies and, above all, to my family, who gave me the strength to see this endeavor through to its conclusion.*

# Preface

Gene therapy, genome editing, and genetic pharmacology are three recent technologies based on the genetic code, which have achieved spectacular and revolutionary therapeutic and vaccine successes since the beginning of the 21st century. They were initially conceived to treat genetic diseases. Most genetic diseases are rare diseases, meaning they affect less than 1 in 2,000 people. There are more than 7,000 of such diseases today, 80% of which are of genetic origin and 95% are incurable. Gene therapy might represent the ultimate solution for these mostly incurable diseases. In the current textbook, the principles of these new therapeutic avenues are described, as well as striking recent clinical successes for rare diseases. These concern, among other examples, lethal and devastating diseases found to be incurable, as well as imperfectly cured diseases such as spinal muscular atrophy, transthyretin amyloidosis, hemoglobinopathies, hemophilia, and dystrophic epidermolysis bullosa.

However, gene therapy has now demonstrated its potency and usefulness not only for rare genetic diseases but also for diseases concerning large numbers of patients, such as cancer, hypercholesterolemia, and COVID-19.

This basic textbook describes the essential concepts and techniques for gene manipulation and gene therapy, as well as a selection of the most striking clinical applications to date. This disruptive and rapidly progressing field has already revolutionized biotechnology, most life sciences, and medicine. The textbook provides a clear and comprehensive description of the technologies currently available for gene delivery, genetic pharmacology, gene therapy, and genome editing. It details the different *in vivo* and *ex vivo* gene delivery and manipulation strategies. It also presents a set of selected biotechnology and therapeutic applications. However, given the exponential growth of this field, a systematic review of all every therapeutic and clinical perspective is beyond the scope of this textbook. Two dedicated chapters (8 and 9) concern of the most recent revolutions: gene editing and personalized adoptive immunotherapy using CAR-T cells.

The two former editions of our *Advanced Textbook on Gene Transfer, Gene Therapy and Genetic Pharmacology* were dedicated to specialized scientists. They represented a compilation of reviews for advanced scientists. The great success of this former advanced textbook and the growing number of gene therapy and genetic pharmacology stakeholders have prompted us to draft a more basic textbook for a larger audience with a general interest in these revolutionary approaches.

The present basic textbook represents a comprehensive description of most of the technologies and applications at the current stage. We hope that it will be of interest and benefit to graduate, advanced undergraduate, and postgraduate students, researchers, physicians, pharmacologists, veterinarians and industry scientists, as well as patients and their organizations. We also hope that our effort will help the readers expand their competencies in the key frontier biological techniques, which are now of critical use in most advanced laboratories everywhere in the world, and encourage them to further deepen their knowledge through the specialized references proposed at the end of each chapter.

# About the Author

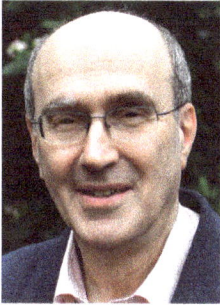

**Daniel Scherman** is Emeritus Research Director at the CNRS National Scientific Research Center and at Université Paris Cité. He has dedicated most of his scientific activity to the gene therapy field, both in terms of delivery methods and for therapeutic applications. He has served several terms in the past and presently on the Scientific Committee of the American Society of Gene and Cell Therapy and as the scientific director of the Généthon Laboratory dedicated to the gene therapy of rare genetic diseases. Professor Daniel Scherman also manages the French Foundation for Rare Diseases.

He is presently the head of the Life Sciences and Medicine Division of the European Academy of Sciences EURASC, and an associated member of the French Academy of Pharmacy.

# Contents

# Part I

# Gene Therapy and Gene Repair

# Chapter 1

# Basic Definitions and General Principles

## 1.1 Definitions

The efficiency of medicinal active agents is based on the universal concept of "target recognition." As stated by Paul Ehrlich in 1913, "In medicinal chemistry, the ruling principle is that active substances are only effective if they have a specific affinity for their target" (in *Chemotherapy*). Ehrlich envisioned that it could be possible to kill specific microbes causing diseases in the body without harming the body itself. This idea led to the development of salvarsan, the first effective drug for syphilis, in 1909. Another key concept in medicinal chemistry had previously been introduced by Emil Fischer in 1894: the "lock and key" concept, which explained enzyme specificity by comparing the enzyme's active site to a lock and the substrate to a key, illustrating how only the correct substrate can initiate a reaction.

The history of medicinal chemistry and biologics is characterized by a limited number of revolutionary advances. Except for traditional medicines derived from the serendipity-driven use of natural plant decoctions, such conceptual revolutions or "quantum leaps" in drug discovery have always resulted from scientific advances.

The first revolution resulted from progress in both analytical and synthetic chemistry, together with Paul Ehrlich's "magic bullet" concept. This has been the basis of the discovery of chemical drugs directed at a molecularly defined "receptor" target. Indeed, before Emil Fischer and Paul Ehrlich's revolutionary ideas, the concept, which is widely accepted today, that molecular receptors in living organisms could be selectively affected by chemical compounds was hardly conceivable.

Biochemistry breakthroughs, along with advances in both protein characterization and recombinant DNA technology, paved the way for the use of proteins as therapeutic agents. Today, recombinant cytokines and hormones, such as erythropoietin (EPO), granulocyte–macrophage colony-stimulating factors (GMCSFs), interferons, and, above all, monoclonal antibodies, represent a considerable achievement and constitute a leading field of drug discovery.

As an overwhelming rule for both chemical and protein drugs, the molecular target in the patient is a protein, with rare exceptions including cytotoxic anticancer agents, such as cisplatin, and a variety of alkylating or intercalating agents, which bind to DNA independently of the genetic sequence.

In contrast to all previous approaches in medicinal chemistry and biologics and representing the most recent revolutionary leap forward, both gene therapy and genetic pharmacology are based on the use of genetic code for target recognition.

In *gene therapy*, presented in Part I, a gene is administered to the patient's cells, leading to the transcription by RNA polymerases of an RNA molecule, which can be by itself a therapeutic agent, or is most often an mRNA molecule translated into a therapeutic protein by the ribosome machinery. In gene therapy, the administered gene can thus be considered a "prodrug," with the amplification advantage resulting from the continuous intracellular production of the therapeutic RNA and, eventually, encoded protein.

Gene therapies, more specifically, refer to the cell delivery of a gene-expressing cassette, namely a transcribed DNA sequence flanked at its 5' end by a eukaryotic promoter and at its 3' end by a polyadenylation signal. This promotes the transcription of an RNA, which either, by itself,

Genomic DNA ◄————————— **Genome editing** corrects Genomic DNA defects *in situ*

**Gene Therapy** delivers a gene flanked by an eukaryotic promoter and a transcription termination signal which leads to the expression of therapeutic RNA or protein

mRNA

**Genetic Pharmacology**: Small oligonucleotides target either DNA or RNA

**Small drug molecules** generally target proteins ————► Protein

**Biologics** are exogenous therapeutic proteins, such as monoclonal antibodies

Function

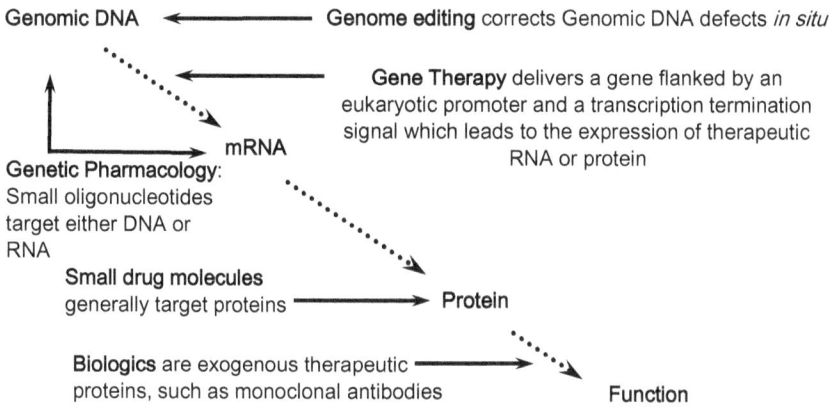

**Figure 1.1.** While chemical drugs classically target proteins (except in the case of anticancer cytotoxic compounds), small chemical oligonucleotides used in genetic pharmacology generally target DNA and/or RNA, with the exception of aptamers. Gene therapy consists of administering a gene-expressing cassette (promoter — gene — polyadenylation signal) to the cells.

displays a therapeutic intracellular effect or encodes a missing protein or any protein or peptide, allowing a therapeutic or vaccination effect. The distinction between genetic pharmacology and gene therapy, as illustrated in Figure 1.1, will be preferentially used in this textbook. However, other authors employ the generic expression "gene therapy" to designate all approaches involving the use of any natural or modified DNA or RNA nucleotide molecules. Examples of potential applications of gene therapy are simply too many to be listed here. Several genetic diseases, which have attracted large interest for gene replacement or genome editing strategies, are presented in Table 1.1 in a non-exhaustive list.

Gene therapy might be used, for instance, to do the following:
- to compensate for a missing protein in a genetic disease;
- to inhibit the production of a given protein (by generating an antisense mRNA), for example to render cells resistant to viral infection;
- to express a trophic factor or an anti-inflammatory cytokine;
- to introduce genetically modified cells, such as anticancer CAR-T cells;
- to introduce a suicide gene or an oncolytic virus for the treatment of cancer.

**Table 1.1.**   Examples of genetic diseases already treated or in clinical trials by gene replacement therapy and their related clinical protocol (a non-exhaustive list).

| Disease | Gene | Clinical protocol |
| --- | --- | --- |
| ADA-SCID immunodeficiency | Adenosine deaminase | *Ex vivo* |
| X-linked immunodeficiency | Gamma-c IL2 receptor subunit | *Ex vivo* |
| Wiskott–Aldrich syndrome | WAS gene | *Ex vivo* |
| Beta-thalassemia | Beta-globin | *Ex vivo* |
| Sickle cell anemia | Beta-globin | *Ex vivo* |
| Hemophilia B | Clotting factor IX | *In vivo* |
| Hemophilia A | Clotting factor VIII | *In vivo* |
| α-1antitrypsin deficiency | α-1 antitrypsin | *In vivo* |
| Duchenne myopathy | Dystrophin | *In vivo* |
| Lipoprotein lipase deficiency | Lipoprotein lipase | *In vivo* |
| **Retinal degenerative disease:** | | |
| Leber congenital amaurosis | RPE 65 (Type 2 LCA) | *In vivo* |
| Stargardt's disease | ABCA4 | *In vivo* |
| X-linked adrenoleukodystrophy | ABCD1 | *Ex vivo* |
| Parkinson's disease | Glutamic acid decarboxylase (GAD) | *In vivo* |
| | Neurturin trophic factor | *In vivo* |
| Lysosomal storage disorders | Lysosomal enzymes | |
| Canavan leukodystrophy | Aspartoacylase | *In vivo* |
| Sanfilippo A (MPSIIIa) | N-sulfoglucosamine sulfohydrolase | *In vivo* |
| Transthyretin amyloidosis | Transthyretin correction | *In vivo* |

*Genome editing*, presented in Chapter 9 of Part I, represents the most recent revolution, in which chromosomal genome abnormalities are directly corrected *in situ* by powerful tools, such as CRISPR-*Cas9*.

*Genetic pharmacology* presented in Part II represents the ultimate step of the "lock and key" concept, in which the drug target is an intracellular genetic sequence within either a DNA or an RNA molecule, which is recognized by Watson–Crick or Hogsteen base pairing. Genetic pharmacology refers to the use of short, synthetic oligonucleotides to manipulate gene expression. This can principally be achieved by the so-called antisense, antigene, or RNA interfering strategies, which will be exemplified in Chapters 10–12.

The specificity of genetic pharmacology, as compared to classical "small chemical drug" pharmacology, is that the short oligonucleotide pharmacological agent recognizes its cognate target through base pairing. The length of the oligonucleotide sequence necessary to ensure target specificity is around 20 bases. The single-strand oligonucleotide (which is either an oligodeoxynucleotide ODN or the antisense strand of a double-strand small interfering RNA — siRNA) generally binds to the mRNA target through Watson–Crick hydrogen bonds, but it can also form a triple helix with DNA duplexes through Hogsteen base pairing. Except for this mechanism of action based on base pair recognition, genetic pharmacology cannot be distinguished from the more classical small drug pharmacology, which is based on receptor-ligand molecular recognition.

## 1.2  Critical Advantages of Gene Therapy

Several fundamental properties render gene therapy essential for the treatment of a large body of diseases, whether genetic or not, and also suggest that it could represent an attractive alternative to protein replacement therapy.

First, since proteins are unable to cross cell membranes, only gene therapy is able to provide for the treatment of any disease which is caused by the lack of expression of an intracellular protein or which can be cured through the intracellular expression of a therapeutic or antigenic protein. This is the case, for instance, with neuromuscular disorders such as Duchenne muscular dystrophy, for which the missing dystrophin protein must be expressed in the muscle cell cytosol. This is also the case for vaccination strategies based on class I antigen presentation.

Second, the delivery of a therapeutic protein leads to temporal variations in its concentration. This can induce toxicity when a transient excessive concentration is observed. Conversely, this can be damaging if the tissue concentration of the missing protein falls below the therapeutic threshold as a result of the short half-life of the administered protein. This deleterious effect of improper patient coverage is observed, for instance, in hemophilia, where patients suffer from severe chronic joint deterioration due to micro-bleeding events occurring at sub-therapeutic threshold concentrations of the replacement clotting factor. The repeated administration of a large dose of the missing clotting factor has been proposed to prevent such damages; however, this has been shown to induce neutralizing antibodies, which inhibit the injected factors.

In contrast to recombinant protein therapy, gene therapy strategy leads to the constant expression of a missing protein when the gene is delivered under the control of a permanently activated promoter, which represents the most frequent case. This important pharmacokinetic advantage of gene therapy, which theoretically allows for "constant coverage" of patients after a single transgene delivery treatment, is illustrated in Figure 1.2.

Another advantage of gene therapy results from the spatial control of its effects. Indeed, by combining the local delivery of a therapeutic transgene and the use of a tissue- or cell-type-specific promoter, one can drastically restrict the expression of the desired protein at a precise location in

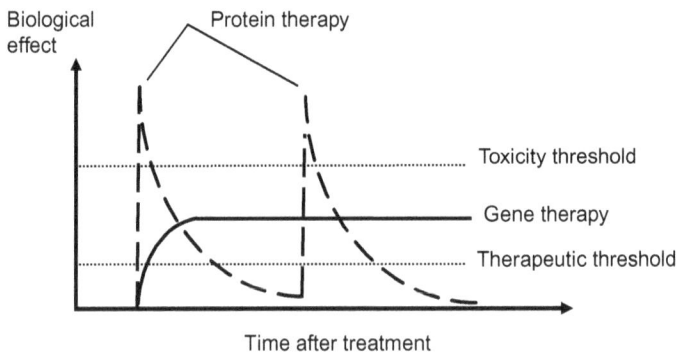

**Figure 1.2.**   Compared pharmacokinetic profiles of protein therapy and gene therapy.

the body of the patient and even in a specific cell type of a given tissue. Such a cell-specific expression has proven to be particularly precious for the treatment of genetic disorders resulting from the complete absence of a protein. An immune response against the missing protein has been observed following gene therapy because the transgenic protein is then considered exogenous by the host patient. By using a cell-type-specific promoter, one can avoid transgene expression in antigen-presenting cells, such as dendritic cells. This results in a decreased immune response against the transgene.

The additional value of cell-type-specific promoters is that they generally lead to a longer and more stable duration of transgene expression, contrary to very strong promoters such as that of the human cytomegalovirus (hCMV), which induce high but transient expression. This is particularly the case in the liver, where the liver-specific alpha-antitrypsin promoter has proven superior to the human cytomegalovirus (hCMV) promoter. In muscle also, studies suggest that the restriction of transgene expression to myotubes is an important criterion for the treatment of muscular dystrophies since it leads to higher and more sustained transgene expression, along with the absence of immune response against the transgene, contrary to what is observed when using the hCMV promoter.

Examples of tissue specific promoters include the following:
- phosphoenolpyruvate carboxykinase (PEPCK) in hepatocytes,
- surfactant protein A (SPA) in epithelial cells (for the treatment of cystic fibrosis),
- desmin (preferentially, skeletal muscle beta-actin, or truncated muscle creatin kinase (MCK) in skeletal muscle cells),
- smooth muscle (SM)-specific SM22α promoter or smooth muscle myosin heavy chain for smooth muscle cells,
- CD11c in dendritic cells,
- glial fibrillary acidic protein (GFAP) in glial cells,
- neuron-specific enolase (NSE) promoter in neurons,
- carcinoembryonic antigen (CEA) promoter for tumor-specific expression.

# 1.3 Temporal Control of Gene Expression

In the context of *in vivo* gene transfer, the temporal regulation of gene expression has a broad range of applications. For example, studying gene function during development often requires gene expression at a particular time. Knocking out these genes (knock-out animals) or overexpressing them (transgenic animals) might result in embryonic lethality, which requires the capacity to express or down-regulate these genes at a specific stage of development. In addition, particularly in the field of gene therapy, a transcriptional regulation system that is rapid, reversible, and repeatedly inducible might be required for safety and efficacy reasons. Several inducible systems in mammalian cells have been developed to artificially regulate genes at the transcriptional level using inducers or repressor small drug molecules.

An ideal gene regulation system has to meet several requirements, particularly the following: (i) high inducibility and low basal level; (ii) no interference with endogenous regulatory networks; and (iii) activation by exogenous, non-toxic drugs of known pharmacology. Early attempts to develop inducible gene expression systems made use of cellular elements that respond to exogenous signals or stress, such as cytokines, hormones, heat, metal ions, and hypoxia. Heat-inducible promoters derived from stress heat-shock proteins and light-switchable promoters based on a stress-related protein have also been developed. These systems are often subject to pleiotropic effects or show high basal activity in the absence of induction. Several artificial systems regulated by a small-molecule inducer (tetracycline, RU486, or ecdysone, for example) have been proposed. The tetracycline-based system, exemplified in Figure 1.3, is the most widely used.

The original tetracycline system (Tet-off) allows for very stringent regulation; however, this system needs permanent tetracyclin or doxycyclin treatment to stop the otherwise constant expression of the transgene. Ideally, a candidate gene therapy system of regulated expression should be an "on" system, where transgene expression is switched on by the administration of a small drug. An alternative version of the Tet system, based

**Regulation of the tetracycline operon**
The Tet repressor is constitutively bound to the TetO operator
The Tet repressor is detached when tetracycline (yellow cross) is added

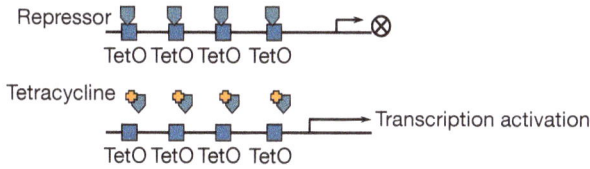

**Tet-off system**
Fusion of the tTA repressor with the HSV-VP16 transactivator leads to transcription
Constitutive transcription activation is terminated by tetracycline addition

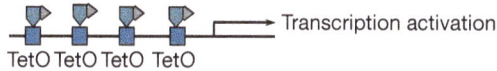

**Tet-on system**
Fusion of the rtTA repressor with VP16 transactivator
Transcription is activated only when tetracycline (yellow cross) binds to the rtTA molecule

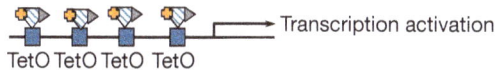

**Figure 1.3.**   Different Tet systems for the temporal control of gene expression. The Tet repressor (green arrow) is constitutively bound to the Tet operator. Tetracycline or docycycline (yellow cross) induce a conformational change, leading to the loss of Tet repressor affinity for the Tet operator DNA sequence. In the Tet-off and Tet-on systems, the VP16 transcriptional activator of the herpes simplex virus (gray triangle) is fused to the Tet repressor or rtTA mutant (hatched white arrow). When bound to DNA, VP16 activates the transcription of the neighboring gene. In the Tet-off system, the presence of tetracycline or doxycycline is necessary to stop gene expression. In the Tet-on system, the addition of tetracycline or doxycycline induces the binding of the reverse tetracyclyne transacticator (rtTA) fused to VP16 to TetO, which leads to VP16-mediated gene transcription, whereas repression depends on the clearance of the antibiotic.

on a mutated form of the tetracycline transactivator (tTA) called reverse tTA (rtTA), has been introduced. The reverse rtTA, which induces transgene expression, binds to DNA only when the small drug inducer is present (Tet-on system).

The major limitations of the Tet-on system in a gene therapy context — particularly important for therapeutic applications — are its poor induction kinetics and high basal level of expression. Therefore, several improvements providing more stringent control of gene expression have been introduced in the form of a mutated transactivator, rtTA2$^S$-M2, or by the addition of the tetracycline transcriptional silencer, tTS.

## 1.4  Codon Optimization

Codon optimization is a technique used to enhance gene expression by modifying the DNA sequence to match the preferred codon usage of host cells.

The principle of codon optimization is based on the redundancy of the genetic code: Several codons can lead to the same amino acid being incorporated into a growing polypeptide chain. For instance, the amino acid alanine is encoded by the codons GCU, GCC, GCA, and GCG; glutamic acid can be encoded by codons GAA and GAG; leucine is encoded by six different codons: UUA, UUG, CUU, CUC, CUA, and CUG; and serine is encoded by the codons UCA, UCG, UCC, UCU, AGU, and AGC. This degeneracy helps to minimize the effects of mutations, as changes in the third position of a codon often do not alter the amino acid being produced.

The concentration of aminoacyl-tRNA varies among the different cell types and organisms and under various stress conditions, and this variability can affect the efficiency and fidelity of protein synthesis, as different cell types may have different demands for specific amino acids and their corresponding tRNAs. Codon optimization aims at inserting into a genetic sequence the codon triplets which correspond to the highest abundance of the corresponding tRNA in the target tissue or cell. This process involves altering the rare codons in the target gene to ensure that the genetic sequence of the transgene more closely reflects the codon usage of the host without changing the amino acid sequence of the encoded protein. This leads to more efficient translation and transgene expression of the desired protein. In addition, codon optimization can improve mRNA stability, thus enhancing transcription and translation efficiency. Codon optimization may also be used to target an immune response toward a specific cell type and tissue. However, some negative side effects of codon optimization have been described, such as alterations in gene expression duration.

## 1.5  Strategies and Protocols for Gene Replacement Therapy, Genome Editing, and Genetic Pharmacology

A large variety of parameters must be selected for each therapeutic approach, as shown in Figure 1.4. These parameters include the following:

*   *Definition of the genetic sequence to be used*: Smaller cDNA sequences are the most frequently used, particularly for viral vectors such as adeno-associated virus (AAV), which have limited encapsidation capacity. On the other hand, genomic sequences or the addition of endogenous introns have been shown to induce a higher, more sustained expression. Codon optimization is frequently used.

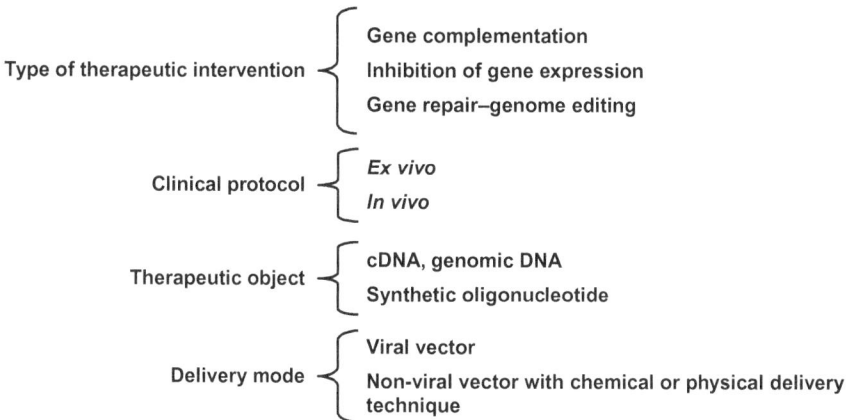

Type of therapeutic intervention
- Gene complementation
- Inhibition of gene expression
- Gene repair–genome editing

Clinical protocol
- *Ex vivo*
- *In vivo*

Therapeutic object
- cDNA, genomic DNA
- Synthetic oligonucleotide

Delivery mode
- Viral vector
- Non-viral vector with chemical or physical delivery technique

**Figure 1.4.**   The definition of a gene therapy protocol necessitates the definition of a panel comprising various parameters. *In vivo* means that the gene therapy drug is administered directly into the body of the patient. *Ex vivo* means that some cells are taken from the patient, modified outside of the patient (*in vitro*), and then readministered to the patient, as shown in Figure 1.5.

- *Duration of transgene expression*: While "burst-type" promoters, such as hCMV, are suitable for genetic vaccination or short-term cytokine expression, tissue-specific promoters might be optimal for "replacement" gene therapy, where long-term expression is needed.
- *Choice of transduction by viral vectors or transfection by non viral vectors*: Integrating vectors, such as retroviral and lentiviral vectors (see Chapter 4), are adapted for transducing stem cells or other dividing cells since integration allows transgene maintenance in daughter cells. Conversely, adenovirus, AAV, herpes viruses, or plasmid non-viral vectors might be more appropriate for gene transfer to differentiated, non-dividing cells. It has to be noted, however, that transposon technology allows plasmid-borne gene chromosomal integration, thereby ensuring transgene maintenance in dividing cells.
- *The required type of genetic intervention*: Gene replacement, gene extinction, or gene repair can be envisioned.
- *The therapeutic protocol*: The therapeutic cassette containing a promoter, the gene of interest (GOI), and a poly(A) tail sequence can be delivered either directly *in vivo* to the patient or *in vitro* to patient-collected cells, which will be subsequently readministered, thus defining an *ex vivo* protocol.

Figure 1.5 illustrates the *in vivo* and *ex vivo* gene therapy protocols. In the *in vivo* case, the therapeutic gene is administered directly to the patient, either as non-viral DNA or mRNA, or borne by a recombinant viral vector, such as an adenovirus, AAV, or herpes virus. In the *ex vivo* protocol, where transgene chromosomal integration into the patient's cells is desired, cells are taken from the patient, gene-modified *in vitro* through either transduction by a recombinant viral vector (such as a recombinant retrovirus or lentivirus) or non-viral transfection using a transposon. The stably modified cells are generally amplified before being readministered to the patient.

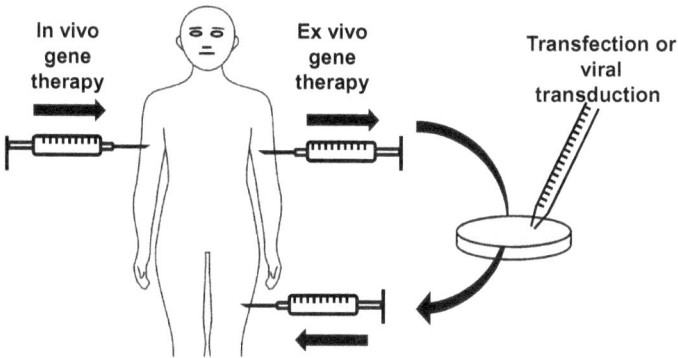

**Figure 1.5.** Scheme of *in vivo* and *ex vivo* gene therapies. In the *in vivo* case, the therapeutic gene is administered directly to the patient either as non-viral DNA or mRNA, or borne by a recombinant viral vector, such as an adenoviral vector, adeno-associated vector (AAV), or recombinant herpes virus. In the *ex vivo* protocol, cells are taken from the patient, gene-modified *in vitro* through either transduction by a recombinant viral vector, such as a retrovirus or lentivirus, or non-viral transfection using a transposon, which leads to transgene chromosomal integration into the patient's cells. The stably modified cells are generally amplified before being readministered to the patient.

# Bibliography

Agha-Mohammadi S, O'Malley M, Etemad A, Wang Z, Xiao X, Lotze MT. Second-generation tetracycline-regulatable promoter: repositioned tet operator elements optimize transactivator synergy while shorter minimal promoter offers tight basal leakiness. *J Gene Med.* 2004 Jul;6(7):817–28. doi: 10.1002/jgm.566.

Curtin JF, Candolfi M, Puntel M, Xiong W, Muhammad AK, Kroeger K, Mondkar S, Liu C, *et al.* Regulated expression of adenoviral vectors-based gene therapies: therapeutic expression of toxins and immune-modulators. *Methods Mol Biol.* 2008;434:239–66. doi: 10.1007/978-1-60327-248-3_15.

Edelmann SL, Nelson PJ, Brocker T. Comparative promoter analysis in vivo: identification of a dendritic cell-specific promoter module. *Blood.* 2011 Sep 15;118(11):e40–9. doi: 10.1182/blood-2011-03-342261. Epub 2011 Jun 9.

Goverdhana S, Puntel M, Xiong W, Zirger JM, Barcia C, Curtin JF, Soffer EB, Mondkar S, *et al.* Regulatable gene expression systems for gene therapy applications: progress and future challenges. *Mol Ther*. 2005 Aug;12(2): 189–211. doi: 10.1016/j.ymthe.2005.03.022.

Núñez-Manchón E, Farrera-Sal M, Otero-Mateo M, Castellano G, Moreno R, Medel D, Alemany R, Villanueva E, *et al*. Transgene codon usage drives viral fitness and therapeutic efficacy in oncolytic adenoviruses. *NAR Cancer*. 2021 Apr 26;3(2):zcab015. doi: 10.1093/narcan/zcab015.

Paremskaia AI, Kogan AA, Murashkina A, Naumova DA, Satish A, Abramov IS, Feoktistova SG, Mityaeva ON, *et al*. Codon-optimization in gene therapy: promises, prospects and challenges. *Front Bioeng Biotechnol*. 2024 Mar 28;12:1371596. doi: 10.3389/fbioe.2024.1371596.

Ribault S, Neuville P, Méchine-Neuville A, Augé F, Parlakian A, Gabbiani G, Paulin D, Calenda V. Chimeric smooth muscle-specific enhancer/promoters: valuable tools for adenovirus-mediated cardiovascular gene therapy. *Circ Res*. 2001 Mar 16;88(5):468–75. doi: 10.1161/01.res.88.5.468.

Talbot GE, Waddington SN, Bales O, Tchen RC, Antoniou MN. Desmin-regulated lentiviral vectors for skeletal muscle gene transfer. *Mol Ther*. 2010 Mar;18(3):601–8. doi: 10.1038/mt.2009.267. Epub 2009 Nov 24.

Weber W, Fussenegger M. Molecular diversity–the toolbox for synthetic gene switches and networks. *Curr Opin Chem Biol*. 2011 Jun;15(3):414–20. doi: 10.1016/j.cbpa.2011.03.003.

# Chapter 2

# Recombinant Viral Vectors: General Considerations

## 2.1 Introduction to Recombinant Viral Vectors

Viruses have been selected by evolution as optimized cell parasites, introducing their genetic material into cells and using the infected cell resources for DNA/RNA replication and protein production for their own expansion. Viruses affect all animals and plants, and also bacteria where they are called phages or bacteriophages. Viruses have developed different potentialities for infecting and replicating in either resting or dividing cells, by introducing their genetic material either as RNA or DNA molecules, in a positive or negative sense with respect to their viral protein coding sequence. This unique capacity to deliver genetic information was from the beginning considered appealing as a gene therapy tool.

A virus-carried genome is either single-stranded (ss) or double-stranded (ds), consisting of two complementary paired nucleic acids. The name of a virus does not correspond to a specific RNA or DNA genome. For instance, different hepatitis viruses, whose names originate from their capacity to preferentially infect liver hepatocytes, can be either RNA or DNA viruses, depending on the type: hepatitis A, C, D, and E are RNA viruses, while hepatitis B virus is a DNA virus (a hepadnavirus).

For most viruses with RNA genomes and some with single-stranded DNA (ssDNA) genomes, the single strand is said to be either positive sense (the "plus strand") or negative sense (the "minus strand"), depending on whether or not it is complementary to the viral messenger RNA (mRNA). Positive-sense viral RNA is in the same sense as viral mRNA, and thus at least a part of it can be immediately translated by the host cell by the ribosome machinery. Negative-sense viral RNA is complementary to mRNA and, therefore, must be converted to positive-sense RNA by an RNA-dependent RNA polymerase before translation. Similarly, positive-strand viral ssDNA is identical in sequence to viral mRNA and is thus a coding strand, while negative-sense viral ssDNA is complementary to viral mRNA and is thus a template strand. Some RNA viral genomes must be retrotranscribed into double-stranded DNA in order to lead to mRNA transcription.

Some viruses have a circular DNA molecule, such as for instance hepatitis B hepadnavirus which has a partially double-stranded and partially single-stranded circular structure. Other viruses have a linear genome, as in the case of adenoviruses (AdVs). The type of nucleic acid is irrelevant to the shape of the genome. Among RNA viruses and certain DNA viruses, the genome is often divided into separate parts, in which case it is called segmented. For RNA viruses, each segment often codes for only one protein and is commonly found together in one capsid. All segments are not required to be in the same virion for the virus to be infectious, as demonstrated by the brome mosaic virus and several other plant viruses.

In a large number of cases, viruses such as AdVs and adeno-associated viruses (AAVs) consist of a viral genome covered by a capsid contained in an assembly of proteins which protects the genome from nucleases and also plays an essential role in recognizing protein receptors on the membranes of the target cells.

Alternatively, several families of viruses, such as the retro- and lentiviruses, herpes virus, flu virus, and COVID-19 virus, are enveloped by an outer membrane. This lipidic membrane contains both viral envelope proteins and components of the infected host cell surface or of endoplasmic reticulum membranes. This viral envelope contains proteins encoded by the viral and host genomes, the lipid membrane itself and any carbohydrates present originate entirely from the host.

## 2.2 General Characteristics of Recombinant Viral Vectors

Gene therapy uses viral vectors to deliver a therapeutic transgene; however, except for oncolytic viruses (see Chapter 3), this must be used as a "one-shot" application. This means that the patient's cells are "transduced" (i.e., they receive genetic material from a viral vector), but they are not "infected", meaning that the virus cannot be replicated and produced by the transduced cells. This constraint has required multiple technological developments for the production of safe "replication-defective" recombinant viruses.

Briefly, replication-defective recombinant viruses are obtained by shearing the viral genome into different parts. Most of the viral genomes are expressed in virus-producing cells, called packaging cells; however, the produced viruses always contain an incomplete, replication-defective, viral genome, in addition to the therapeutic gene of interest. The viral genes are mostly brought by transfection of genetic material. In this *in vitro* transfection step, the viral genes are delivered as plasmids to the packaging cells by using the chemical or physical delivery techniques described in Chapters 6 and 7. In some cases, however, the packaging cell line might have been optimized through stable chromosomal insertion of essential viral proteins devoid of toxicity for these cells. In all scenarios, the viral proteins are expressed *in trans*, meaning that they are produced by the packaging cells, but their corresponding viral genetic sequences are not incorporated into the produced recombinant viral vector. Thus, the genome inserted in the viral vectors is devoid of viral sequences, except those necessary for encapsidation and, in the case of retro- and lentiviruses, those necessary for chromosomal integration into the patient's cells.

For AdVs, the transfection of a single recombinant AdV plasmid into a packaging cell is sufficient to produce recombinant AdV particles (see Chapter 3). For other viral vector productions, such as AAVs and retro-/lentiviral vectors, the essential viral protein genes are inserted into two or three independent plasmids (Chapters 3 and 4). These viral genome plasmids contain the sequence of essential viral proteins and are devoid of encapsidation sequences, thus avoiding the packaging of viral genes into the recombinant viral vector. In addition, a "shuttle vector" contains the recombinant therapeutic expression cassette, consisting of an eukaryotic promoter, the therapeutic gene of interest (GOI), and a poly(A) sequence. This therapeutic plasmid contains the sequences necessary for GOI incorporation into the viral vector. These sequences are the inverted terminal repeats (ITRs) for AdVs and AAVs and the psi (Ψ) sequences for retro- and lentiviruses.

The most widely used packaging cell lines are derived from the HEK293 cell line, which originates from human embryonic kidney cells. For AdV, AAV, or lentiviral gene therapy vectors, transient transfection of HEK293T cells is generally used. These cells were modified from HEK293 to include the SV40 large T-antigen, which enhances their ability to produce high levels of recombinant proteins and viruses.

While retroviral- or lentiviral-derived recombinant vectors are collected in the HEK293T cell culture supernatant, the lysis of packaging cells is required to release mature AdV or AAV particles that are trapped within the packaging cells. Cell lysis can be achieved through various methods, such as freeze/thaw cycles, chemical lysis, or mechanical disruption. Purification is achieved through various techniques, including gradient centrifugation and affinity chromatography using immobilized antibodies. One of the strongest challenges in the production of very high titers of recombinant viruses is the complete elimination of replication-competent viral particles. This imposes stringent optimization of the production process and drastic quality control at the end of the production before the delivery of a clinical batch.

The desired duration of expression of the transgene introduced into the target cells may vary depending on each therapeutic application. Short-term expression is adequate for treating acute conditions, such as cardiac injuries, or for vaccine applications, while long-term expression may be required to treat chronic conditions. Long-term expression can be achieved in non-dividing cells by a DNA virus delivered into the nucleus, preferentially in an episomal circular form, as by, for instance, an AAV vector.

Because the episomal viral genome is lost upon cell division, genome-integrating viruses are necessary for stable expression in dividing cells. This is the case for T-lymphocytes genetically modified to express a chimeric antigen receptor (CAR-T cells, Chapter 8) and, generally, when gene therapy is performed on hematopoietic stem cells. In such cases, recombinant defective retroviruses and lentiviruses have been used since they possess the capacity to integrate their retrotranscribed genome into the host genome by using their integrase protein. While retroviruses realize this integration process only in dividing cells, this is not the case with lentiviruses, such as the human immunodeficiency virus (HIV-1), which possesses the interesting capacity to integrate its retrotranscribed genome into both dividing and non-dividing cells.

## 2.3 Packaging Capacity and Tropism

An important aspect is the limited packaging capacity of a recombinant viral vector, which is linked to a quite constrained structural capacity of the capsid of non-enveloped viruses or that of the core (also known as the nucleocapsid) of enveloped viruses. A critical point is the low packaging capacity of AAV vectors (<5 kilobases, or kb). For instance, while several AAV serotypes have been shown to highly efficiently transduce muscle cells, their limited packaging capacity precludes them from delivering integral cDNA of the dystrophin gene, which is mutated in patients affected by Duchenne muscular dystrophy and has a size of approximately 14 kb. This has fostered research into functional truncated forms of the dystrophin protein, the so-called mini-dystrophin or micro-dystrophin, in order to accommodate the 5 kb size limit. In such a strategy, it is necessary to precisely identify the parts of the protein required for function and to verify that deletion of certain segments still maintains a functional three-dimensional structure.

Alternative techniques have been proposed to solve the AAV limited capacity problem, such as producing two different AAV vectors, each carrying one part of the therapeutic gene, while taking advantage of intracellular mRNA trans-splicing to assemble in the transduced cells a fully functional complete protein. Also, other viral vectors such as herpes simplex 1 (HSV-1) or retroviral and lentiviral recombinant vectors possess a higher packaging capacity. This has been used for the recently approved gene therapy for a very severe skin condition, epidermolysis bullosa, in which an HSV-1 vector is used to deliver the 9 kb collagen 7A1 cDNA.

Another important factor is the capacity for a recombinant virus to transduce the desired patient cells, which is strictly dependent on the virus' tropism. For this reason, human viruses have been the most investigated and used, although murine, monkey, or canine viruses have also proven effective as potent viral vectors for delivering genetic payloads to human cells. An "amphotropic" virus is a type of virus that can infect and replicate in a wide range of host species and cell types. Unlike some viruses that have a very narrow host range ("ecotropic" viruses), amphotropic viruses can recognize receptors on cells from different species and cell types, and efficiently transduce them. A broad host range is appealing for gene therapy applications. However, in some cases, the restriction to a specific cell type may be required because the expressed transgene could have detrimental effects on other cell types. In such cases, ecotropic viruses might be preferential. The genome of recombinant viral vectors has been extensively manipulated to either extend or restrict their tropism. These non-natural viruses, in which the capsid or envelope proteins have been modified to specifically recognize certain human cell receptors, are called "pseudotyped" viruses. Some examples are presented in Chapters 3 and 4.

Table 2.1 summarizes some properties of the most commonly used gene therapy recombinant viral vectors and their clinical use. AdV, AAV, and HSV-1 recombinant viruses are administered *in vivo* to patients. Some attempts have also been made to deliver retro- and lentiviral vectors *in vivo*, for instance in brain tissue. However, retroviral and lentiviral recombinant viral vectors are mainly used through an *ex vivo* procedure, in which autologous cells are taken from the patient, stably transduced *in vitro*, and subsequently readministered to the patient.

**Table 2.1.** Characteristics of the most commonly used viral gene therapy vectors.

| Viral vector clinical use | Genetic material | Packaging capacity | Host range | Limitations or safety concern |
|---|---|---|---|---|
| Adenovirus *In vivo* | dsDNA | 8 kb (replication defective) 30 kb (helper dependent) | Broad | Inflammatory response |
| AAV *In vivo* | ssDNA or scDNA (ds) | <5 kb | Broad (serotype dependent) | Small packaging capacity |
| Retrovirus *Ex vivo* | RNA | 8 kb | Broad | Only transduces dividing cells Risk of insertional oncogenesis |
| Lentivirus *Ex vivo* | RNA | 8 kb | Restricted  Broad when pseudotyped | Can transduce non-dividing cells Risk of insertional oncogenesis |
| HSV-1 *In vivo* | dsDNA | 40 kb (replication defective) 150 kb (amplicon) | Broad | Inflammatory response Transient gene expression in non-neuronal cells |

## 2.4 General Challenges to Recombinant Viral Vectors

Replication-defective recombinant viruses represent highly efficient gene delivery vectors, and the availability of various viruses allows for selecting the one best suited for each therapeutic application. In many cases, several different viruses can achieve a similar gene delivery function, and so various parallel strategies are pursued. Consequently, recombinant viral vectors are increasingly entering into routine clinical use, such as lentiviral vectors for CAR-T cell production and AAVs for liver metabolic disorders and eye diseases.

However, several key issues remain that continue to limit the generalization of the use of recombinant viral vectors. The following are several problems that have appeared during the course of viral gene therapy development, which remain to be better mastered: (1) temporal control of transgene expression; (2) selective and efficient *in vivo* targeting and delivery to the required tissue/organ; (3) immune response against the viral vector and the transgene; (4) associated toxicity, especially hepatotoxicity; (5) insertional oncogenesis by integrative vectors; (6) limited packaging capacity; and (7) limitations in bioproduction capacity.

(1) *Temporal control of transgene expression*: Gene therapy, ideally, represents a "one shot for life" curative solution. Although this may be desirable for chronic diseases, it is necessary in certain cases or when an acute toxic effect occurs to stop the treatment. Temporal control of gene expression systems are available for animal experiments, but not approved yet for clinical use. The rapid development of mRNA drugs delivered by non-viral techniques might represent an attractive solution due to their short cellular half-life.

(2) *Selective and efficient in vivo targeting and delivery to the required tissue/organ*: Proper *in vivo* targeting of the required tissue/organ, crossing the blood–brain barrier to transduce efficiently large regions of the brain, and de-targeting virus entry into unwanted cells such as dendritic cells to limit immune response or into liver cells to control hepatotoxicity all represent important challenges. Also, it is still not possible to efficiently transduce tissues, such as pulmonary epithelium or digestive tract epithelium, which would be of great value for treating cystic fibrosis and other diseases through gene therapy.

(3) *Immune response against the viral vector and the transgene*: The host immune system can recognize and neutralize the recombinant viral vector, thereby reducing its effectiveness and potentially causing adverse reactions. Pre-existing neutralizing antibodies preclude the use of certain AAV

serotypes in some patient populations. Also, the buildup of a strong, lasting immune response against a recombinant viral vector, such as an AAV, makes it impossible to use the same AAV serotype twice in a single patient. Hence, for chronic diseases, if the expression of the therapeutic gene weakens over time, it is not possible to apply the same gene therapy protocol more than once. Also, in a gene replacement therapy context, the transduced wild-type gene leads to the expression of a protein which is normally absent from the patient and is thus recognized as a foreign protein. This triggers an immune response against the cells expressing the therapeutic proteins, which must be controlled. Strategies to avoid transducing immune competent cells, such as dendritic cells, are considered in this context, for instance by placing the transgene under the control of a promoter inactive in dendritic cells.

(4) *Associated toxicity, especially hepatotoxicity*: For the clinically approved AAV gene therapy administered to the liver of patients with clotting disorders, heavy corticotherapy is required for between several weeks and several months, sometimes even consisting of long-term corticotherapy, which can induce side effects such as weight gain, hypertension, diabetes, osteoporosis, and increased risk of infections. These risks, associated with the fact that gene therapy in hemophilia patients might not be fully curative for a large proportion of patients, are hampering the acceptance of this revolutionary treatment among the hemophilia community. Corticotherapy is necessary because of the immune response against the viral vector or transgene expressed in the liver. Hepatotoxicity is the most common adverse event observed with high doses of adenoviral or AAV vectors. Although mild in most cases, hepatotoxicity may affect gene therapy efficacy and lead to acute liver failure, persistent hepatitis necessitating prolonged use of immunosuppressants, and, in some rare cases, death. Some of these acute hepatotoxic adverse events might be related not only to an immune response against the vector or transgene but also to a specific disease-related susceptibility. This seems to be the case for the rare gentic disorder myotubular myopathy. Thus, although gene therapy applications of AAV vectors are generally considered safe, the administration in

the blood systemic circulation of high vector doses, which are required, for instance, for muscular disorders in which a large amount of tissue has to be transduced, can lead to uncontrolled severe side effects. Potentially fatal outcomes in individual patients have been observed, especially after activation of the immune system, which fosters the identification of new and potent methods for immunosuppression, the reduction of AAV dose, or the use of alternative, less immunogenic vectors. In summary, there is an urgent need for empiric protocols to diagnose and treat hepatotoxicity, which would be based on the side-effect profile of individual gene therapy, our present understanding of the immunological basis of hepatotoxicity, previous experience with various immunosuppressants in other disorders, and the unique challenges and requirements of gene therapy.

(5) *Insertional oncogenesis by integrative vectors*: Insertional oncogenesis, observed with integrative vectors, has led to cancer occurrence in several patients. With the development of self-inactivating SIN-retroviral and SIN-lentiviral vectors, this risk is now reasonably controlled (see Chapter 4). However, research is still needed to efficiently target transgene integration into so-called genomic "safe harbors", where no oncolytic event can be anticipated.

(6) *Limited packaging capacity*: Limited packaging capacity of AAVs and retro-/lentiviral vectors still represents a barrier for certain applications. In particular, the so-called self-complementary scAAV vectors, although showing some advantages in terms of rapidity of transgene expression, have half the packaging capacity of standard AAVs, further limiting the size of the genetic material they can carry.

(7) *Limitations in bioproduction capacity*: Limitations in bioproduction capacity represent an important bottleneck. Manufacturing and purifying high-quality vectors at a large scale can be complex and costly; it also remains unsolved for treating large tissue masses, such as those found in muscle diseases. To achieve large-scale production, researchers have

developed processes using baculovirus expression vectors in insect cell cultures. Additionally, vectors are produced by cells in suspension without animal-derived components. Still, the large amount of viral doses required to fulfill patient needs actually preclude treating a large number of patients, as both global production capacity and the very high associated costs are limiting factors.

These many challenges highlight the need for ongoing research and development to optimize viral vectors for gene therapy applications.

# Bibliography

Aiuti A, Pasinelli F, Naldini L. Ensuring a future for gene therapy for rare diseases. *Nat Med.* 2022 Oct;28(10):1985–1988. doi: 10.1038/s41591-022-01934-9.

Arjomandnejad M, Dasgupta I, Flotte TR, Keeler AM. Immunogenicity of recombinant adeno-associated virus (AAV) vectors for gene transfer. *BioDrugs.* 2023 May;37(3):311–329. doi: 10.1007/s40259-023-00585-7.

Dobrowsky T, Gianni D, Pieracci J, Suh J. AAV manufacturing for clinical use: insights on current challenges from the upstream process perspective. *Current Opinion in Biomedical Engineering.* 2021 Dec;20(20):100353. doi. org/10.1016/j.cobme.2021.100353.

Dunbar CE. A plethora of gene therapies for hemoglobinopathies. *Nat Med.* 2021 Feb;27(2):202–204. doi: 10.1038/s41591-021-01235-7.

Ghosh S, Brown AM, Jenkins C, Campbell K. Viral vector systems for gene therapy: a comprehensive literature review of progress and biosafety challenges. *Appl Biosaf.* 2020 Mar;25(1):7–18. doi: 10.1177/1535676019899502.

Horn S, Fehse B. How safe is gene therapy? Second death after Duchenne therapy. *Inn Med.* 2024 Jun;65(6):617–623. doi: 10.1007/s00108-024-01711-5.

Hosseinkhani H, Domb A, Sharifzadeh G, Nahum. Gene therapy for regenerative medicine. *Pharmaceutics.* 2023;15:856. https://doi.org/10.3390/pharmaceutics15030856.

Jagadisan B, Dhawa A. Hepatotoxicity in adenoassociated viral vector gene therapy. *Current Hepatology Reports.* 2023;22:276–290. https://doi.org/10.1007/s11901-023-00624-5.

Kilgore R, Minzoni A, Shastry S, Smith W, Barbieri E, Wu Y, LeBarre JP, Chu W, *et al*. The downstream bioprocess toolbox for therapeutic viral vectors. *J Chromatogr A*. 2023 Oct;1709:464337. doi: 10.1016/j.chroma. 2023.464337.

Ronzitti G, Gross DA, Mingozzi F. Human immune responses to adeno-associated virus (AAV) vectors. *Front Immunol*. 2020 Apr;11:670. doi: 10.3389/ fimmu.2020.00670.

# Chapter 3

# Episomal Non-Integrative Viral Vectors: AdV, AAV, and HSV-1

## 3.1 Adenoviral Vectors

Human adenoviruses (AdVs) can cause a variety of diseases, including infections of the respiratory and the digestive tracts and conjunctivitis. Recombinant replication-defective adenoviral vectors possess the capability to transduce a large variety of cells. Their large genome allows the insertion of long genes of interest, especially the second- and third-generation (gutless) adenoviral vectors, from which most of the viral genome has been deleted.

AdVs are large (~950 Å) and complex non-enveloped viruses. They contain a linear double-stranded DNA (dsDNA) genome, and their capsid displays icosahedral symmetry. At least 12 different proteins compose the virion. These include the major and minor capsid proteins, core proteins, maturation protease, terminal protein, and packaging machinery. Several minor coat proteins help to assemble and maintain the shell. Three of them (IIIa, VI, and VIII) are conserved throughout the entire adenoviridae family and are therefore expected to play crucial roles during assembly. Protein VI is a key factor for AdV entry into the host cell, following attachment mediated by the penton base and fiber.

The penton base and the spike fiber are essential components of the AdV structure. The penton base is a pentameric protein located at the summit of the icosahedral capsid, to which the fiber is attached. Both penton base and fiber play a significant role in the virus' ability to attach to and enter host cells. The fiber interacts with the coxsackievirus and Adenovirus Receptor (CAR) on the host cell surface. This receptor is a transmembrane protein that serves as an initial attachment point for coxsackieviruses and AdVs. The CAR is encoded in humans by the CXADR gene, and it is expressed in various tissues, including the heart, brain, and epithelial and endothelial cells, hence conferring the amphotropic character of adenoviral vectors.

After the initial attachment to the CAR receptor, the penton base AdV coat protein, which contains the peptide motif arginyl-glycyl-aspartic acid (RGD), binds to the integrin cell surface receptors $\alpha v \beta 3$ and $\alpha v \beta 5$ (Figure 3.1). Binding to these cell surface integrins induces AdV cellular

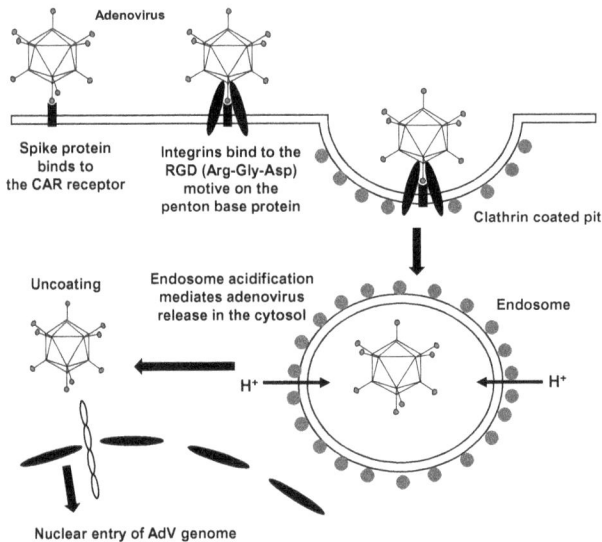

**Figure 3.1.**    AdV entry into the cells. Binding of the fiber to the CAR receptor represents the first cell membrane attachment step. Then, integrins $\alpha v \beta 3$ and $\alpha v \beta 5$ bind to the penton base, and this promotes AdV endocytosis into clathrin-coated pits (gray circles represent clathrin molecules). Endosome acidification induces conformational changes in AdV capsid proteins, causing endosomal lysis and release of the AdV particle into the cytosol. The destabilized AdV capsid uncoats in the cytosol, and the released double-stranded DNA is transported to the nucleus through the nuclear pores.

internalization into early endosomal compartments via clathrin-coated pits. Subsequent endosomal acidification, linked to the activity of the endosomal proton-pump ATPase, causes conformational changes in capsid proteins, which leads to endosomal escape, thus avoiding lysosomal degradation of viral particles. The protein involved in AdV endosomal escape is protein VI, which is responsible for inducing membrane damage following a pH-dependent conformational change.

After this endosomal leakage step, AdV vectors travel through microtubules to the nuclear membrane. Upon capsid disassembly, the viral genome is imported into the nucleus through the nuclear pore complexes, involving nucleoporins such as Nup214 and Nup358. The viral genome is then released into the nucleus, allowing transcription and translation of the therapeutic gene.

The production of a replication-defective recombinant AdV vector is illustrated in Figure 3.2. A single recombinant adenoviral plasmid is transfected into HEK293T packaging cells. Other cell lines derived from HEK293 have been used for specific viral vectors, such as the AD293 cells, which contain a genomic integration of several AdV type 5 genetic sequences. These HEK293-derived cells are particularly useful in research for producing recombinant AdV particles because they produce the AdV E1 protein *in trans*, allowing the production of AdV virus particles when transfected with E1-deleted AdV vectors.

The AdV E1 gene, specifically the E1A region, is one of the first genes expressed during AdV infection. It plays a crucial role in the viral life cycle by producing proteins that help the virus replicate and modulate the host cell's environment, such as stimulating the host cell to enter the S cell cycle phase, creating an environment favorable to viral replication, or enhancing or repressing the expression of both viral and cellular genes. Since the E1 gene is essential for efficient virus replication, the deletion of the E1 gene from adenoviral vectors renders the virus replication-incompetent, which is necessary for creating safe gene therapy vectors.

While first-generation AdV vectors were only deleted from E1 and, to some extent, from the E3 gene, second-generation AdV vectors have been created to further increase viral gene deletions in the recombinant vector

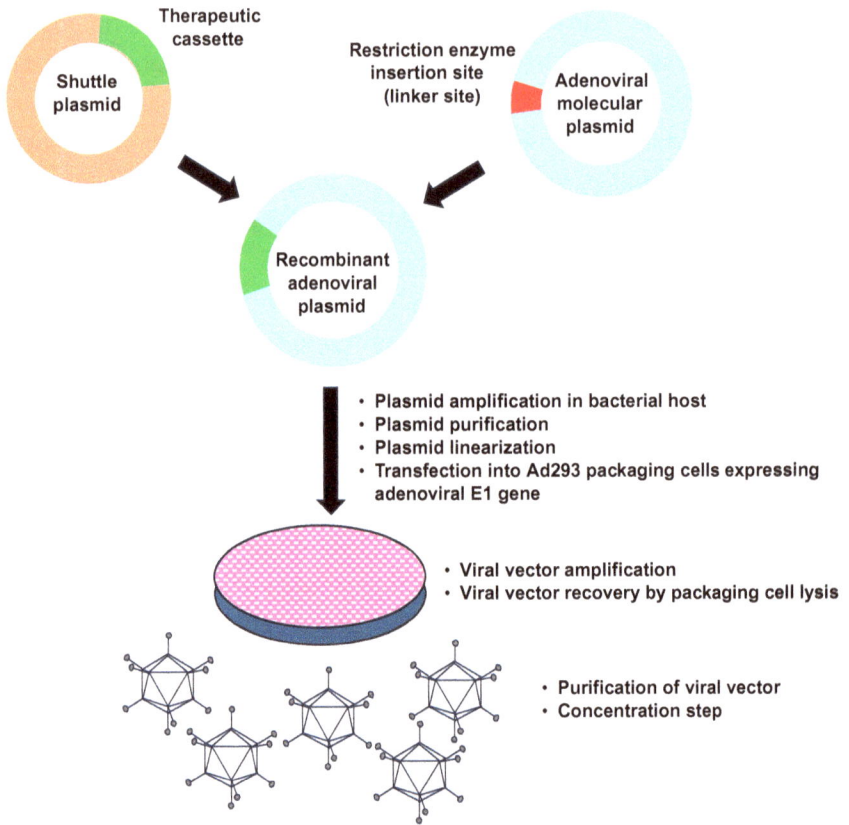

**Figure 3.2.** AdV vector production. A recombinant expression cassette containing a eukaryotic promoter, the gene of interest, and a poly(A) sequence is inserted into a "shuttle" plasmid. A second plasmid contains AdV genes, except for the E1 (ΔE1 AdV genome). These two plasmids are used as a source to create a recombinant AdV plasmid that contains the therapeutic cassette inserted between AdV ITRs, which are necessary for initiating genome replication and packaging the viral genome into the capsid. The recombinant AdV plasmid is devoid of critical adenoviral sequences, such as the E1 gene. It is transfected into a virus-producing cell using non-viral chemical or physical techniques, as described in Chapters 6 and 7. First-generation AdV vectors are deleted from either the early (E) region 1 (E1) or the E1 and E3 regions of the viral genome. Deletion of the E1 region results in a replication-incompetent vector, and it also increases the size of the therapeutic cassette, which can be carried by the AdV vector. E1-deleted AdV vectors can only grow in a cell line (e.g., HEK 293) that constitutively expresses E1 proteins.

(ΔE2 and ΔE4). In the most recent third generation of AdV vectors, all viral genes are removed, but these "gutless" AdVs require the concomitant use of a helper vector carrying the AdV genes, which is co-transfected in the HEK293T packaging cells, together with the plasmid containing the therapeutic cassette and the two inverted terminal repeats (ITRs).

The main existing and prospective clinical applications of adenoviral vectors concern multiple recombinant vaccines and cancer treatments (see the section on oncolytic viruses). An interesting application is that of *nadofaragene firadenovec* (Adstiladrin), which is a gene therapy for the treatment of non-muscle invasive bladder cancer unresponsive to BCG (Bacillus Calmette-Guérin). This gene therapy drug consists of an AdV vector that encodes interferon IFN-$\alpha$2b. It represents the first approved gene therapy for bladder cancer. The production of IFN-$\alpha$2b by transduced urothelial cells is associated with anticancer activity, including immunostimulatory, antiangiogenic, and apoptotic effects. This drug was approved by the FDA in 2022 for the treatment of high-risk, BCG-unresponsive non-muscle invasive bladder cancer *in situ* with or without papillary tumors, in adults. Signaling mediated by IFN-$\alpha$ is involved in the stimulation of anticancer immune responses, which ultimately include the activation of dendritic cells and subsequent priming of cytotoxic T cells and natural killer cells against cancer. The gene therapy drug is administered through the intravesical route (for bladder cancer), with development using intrapleural injections for mesotheliomas.

## 3.2 Adeno-Associated Viral Vectors

The adeno-associated viruses (AAVs) are small DNA viruses of the family Parvoviridae, whose three viral capsid proteins (VP1, VP2, and VP3) form a non-enveloped shell of icosahedral symmetry. The AAVs possess wide tissue tropism. They present low pathogenicity, mainly because they rely on a "helper" virus for their replication, which in gene therapy protocols is an adenovirus. Thus, recombinant AAV vectors display an additional level of biosafety. These favorable characteristics have fostered intense development, and recombinant AAV (rAAV) has already been approved for several gene therapy indications, with many more to come.

The AAV genome is linear. It consists of single-stranded DNA (ssDNA), which is approximately 4.7 kb long. Hence, in the natural process of AAV intracellular biology, the synthesis of a complementary DNA strand is necessary, which might slow down and decrease the efficacy of transgene expression. To circumvent this difficulty, a self-complementary adeno-associated virus (scAAV) was introduced. It is a recombinant viral vector engineered from the naturally occurring AAV. Unlike the standard AAV, which has a single-stranded DNA genome, the scAAV has a dsDNA genome. This design allows for faster and more efficient gene expression because it bypasses the need for the host cell to synthesize the complementary DNA strand. However, the scAAV has a reduced packaging capacity compared to the standard AAV, which reduces the size of the genetic material it can package and deliver by a factor of two.

A typical production scheme of a recombinant AAV vector is displayed in Figure 3.3. It uses the co-transfection of three different plasmids. The first plasmid contains the therapeutic expression cassette, flanked by two ITR sequences. The AAV vectors' ITRs play a crucial role in the life cycle of the virus and its function as a gene therapy vector. They are essential for packaging the viral genome into the AAV capsid since the DNA sequence between the ITRs is the one that is packaged into the AAV vector. The ITRs also help convert the single-stranded AAV genome into a double-stranded form, which is necessary for the transcription and expression of the transgene.

The second co-transfected plasmid contains the AAV genes Rep and Cap, encoding the proteins replicase, Rep, and capsid, Cap, which play essential roles in its life cycle and functionality as a gene therapy vector. They are involved in several critical functions: Rep proteins (Rep78, Rep68, Rep52, and Rep40) are necessary for the replication of the AAV genome into a dsDNA; they regulate the transcription of AAV genes, including the cap gene, and help in packaging the viral genome into the capsid. The Rep proteins also facilitate the integration of the wild-type AAV genome into the host genome at a specific site on human

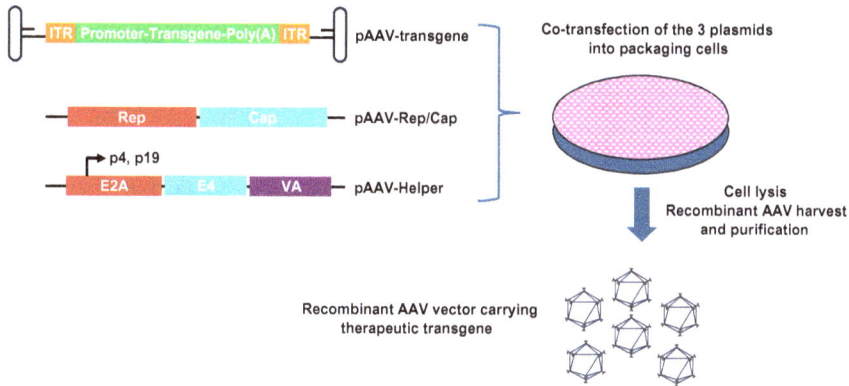

**Figure 3.3.** Production of a recombinant AAV vector implying the co-transfection of three plasmids. The role of the different genetic sequences is described in the text. The AAV ITRs are essential for gene encapsidation. Since only the therapeutic transgene is flanked by the ITRs, it will be the only one encased within the recombinant viral vector. Thus, the recombinant viral vector rAAV has transduction capacity but is not infective; it cannot be replicated after delivery into the patient's cells.

chromosome 19; however, it does so with low efficiency. This unwanted integration capacity has been considered negligible in current gene therapy protocols.

The Cap proteins (VP1, VP2, and VP3) are structural components of the AAV capsid; they are involved in encapsidating the AAV genome and also determining the tropism of the virus because they are the ones that bind to cellular receptors. This means they determine which types of cells the virus can infect so that genetic modifications of these proteins can be attempted in order to increase AAV tissue or cell selectivity. Such genetic modifications, however, are limited by the constraints linked to capsid assembly, stability, virus endosomal leakage, and capsid disassembly.

The third co-transfected plasmid contains the helper genes consisting of adenoviral E2A, EA, and VA genes. The E2A gene encodes a DNA-binding protein which plays a crucial role in AAV DNA replication, transcription, and host cell metabolism. The AdV E2A protein helps mediate AAV replication by activating the AAV p5 and p19 promoters, thereby controlling the expression of the AAV Rep proteins. The E4 protein enhances AAV DNA replication and late viral protein synthesis, and it inhibits the formation of viral genome concatemers. It promotes AAV second-strand synthesis and prevents the degradation of AAV capsids and the Rep52 protein. The viral associated (VA) gene in the AdV helper genome encodes for VA RNA, a type of non-coding RNA that regulates translation within the packaging cells. There are two copies of this RNA, known as VAI (VA RNAI) and VAII (VA RNAII).

During the manufacturing process, cell lysis is a key downstream operation, where the packaging cell membrane is broken down to release the viral vector from the host cell. Purification is achieved through various methods, including cesium chloride gradient centrifugation, dialysis, and immune-affinity chromatography. One of the goals of the cesium chloride gradient centrifugation is to separate genuine transgene-loaded rAAV particles with transduction capacity from empty AAV capsids. These empty capsids have no therapeutic effect and are deleterious in terms of enhancing the immune response against the vector.

AAV families are defined by their serotype, meaning their recognition by specific antibodies that bind to their capsid. Currently, 12 AAV serotypes (designated as AAV1–AAV12) have been identified with variable tropism, and over 100 AAV variants have been isolated from human/nonhuman primate tissues. The serotypes AAV2, AAV3, AAV5, and AAV6 have been discovered in human cells, while the serotypes AAV1, AAV4, AAV7, AAV8, AAV9, AAV10 (AAVrh10), AAV11, and AAV12 have been found in non-human primate samples, such as AAVrh10 in rhesus monkey.

AAV viruses and recombinant viral vectors infect or transduce host cells through a multi-step process (Figure 3.4):

(1) Attachment to specific cell surface receptors on the host cell through interaction with VP1, VP2, or VP3, which form the outer shell of the virus capsid: Different AAV serotypes use different receptors for cell binding. For example, AAV2 binds to heparan sulfate proteoglycan on the cell membrane, AAV5 interacts with sialic acid moieties, and AAV9 utilizes terminal N-linked galactose for cellular entry. These interactions are crucial for the virus' ability to transduce specific cell types.

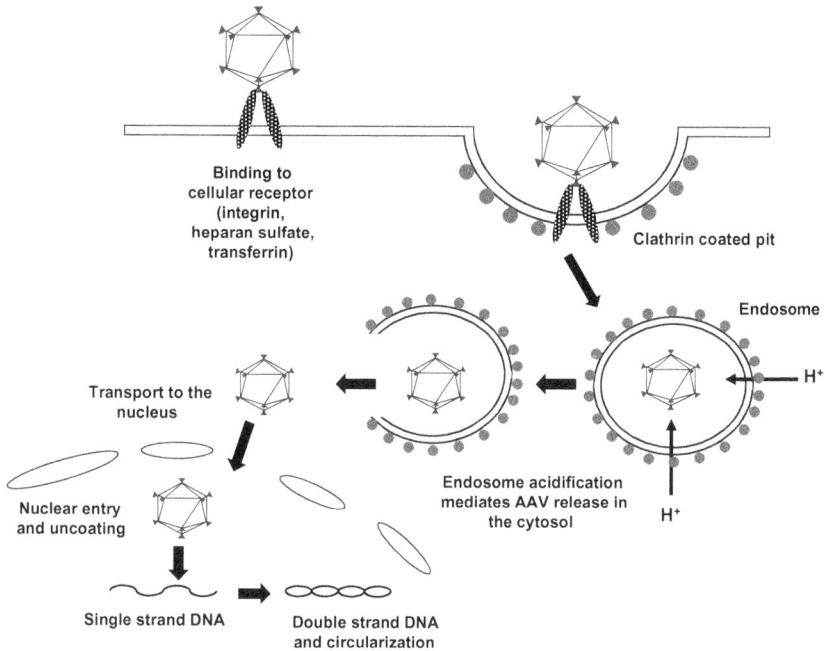

**Figure 3.4.** AAV entry into the cells. Integrin α5β1 has been identified as a coreceptor for AAV2 infection. This interaction is mediated by a highly conserved domain in the AAV2 capsid, which contains an asparagine-glycine-arginine (NGR) motif. Other serotypes bind to heparan sulfate proteoglycan or the transferrin receptor. After acidic-pH-mediated release from the endosome, AAVs are transported to the nucleus of the transduced cell. They uncoat and release their genetic material in the nucleus. The uncoating process is stepwise and involves structural reorganization within the nucleolus.

(2) Internalization into the cell via endocytosis.

(3) Endosomal escape: Once inside the cell, AAVs escape from the endosome into the cytoplasm. This process occurs through conformational changes of viral capsid proteins in the endosomal acidic compartment. The AAV capsid protein, responsible for endosomal escape in an acidic environment, is primarily VP1 but also includes VP2. The acidic pH induces a conformational change that exposes several domains in the N-termini of VP1 and VP2, which are usually buried inside the capsid. These domains assist the AAV virion in escaping from the endosomal-lysosomal system.

(4) AAV transport to the nucleus of the host cell.
(5) AAV uncoating, and ssDNA used as a template for dsDNA synthesis and circularization.

The AAV tropism is mainly dependent on its serotype. It has been observed that several hypervariable regions of the virus capsid are responsible for specific cell tropism. This versatility has been further enhanced by the introduction of rAAV vectors containing custom-engineered capsids with modifications to the VP1, VP2, and VP3 capsid proteins, as mentioned above. Such capsid engineering toward chimeric AAV vectors presents a great potential for gene therapy applications and requires techniques such as DNA shuffling, error-prone PCR, and directed point mutations to evolve the natural capsid proteins. An example of this is the clinically approved AAVrh74, which displays an interesting capacity for targeting muscle cells; it is further described at the end of this section.

A general method of developing new AAVs with improved selectivity and lower toxicity involves decreasing the natural liver tropism, which is associated with severe adverse events at high dosages that might be necessary for achieving therapeutic transgene expression in extrahepatic tissues. Capsid engineering can be achieved by generating AAV libraries containing variations at the VP1 protein. For example, three residues (Y446, N470, and W503) of the galactose-binding pocket of the AAV9 VP1 protein were systematically modified. Screening of this library for *in vivo* tropism in mice identified a family of variants that exhibited significantly reduced liver RNA expression and increased cardiac RNA expression when compared to the wild-type AAV9. In such studies, however, species specificities must be taken into account.

Some key aspects of the most commonly used serotypes of AAV gene therapy vectors are summarized in the following, with examples of clinically approved drugs, which all involve *in vivo* vector delivery.

**AAV2** is the first described AAV isolate and also the best-studied AAV serotype. In addition to heparan sulfate proteoglycan, two coreceptors — $\alpha V \beta 5$ integrin and fibroblast growth factor (FGF) receptor — participate in AAV entry into cells through receptor-mediated endocytosis.

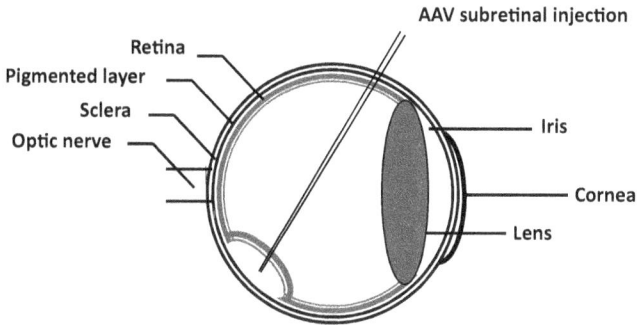

**Figure 3.5.** Subretinal injection of AAV2 carrying the RPE65 gene for treatment of RPE65-related retinal dystrophy. The retinal pigment epithelium-specific 65 kDa protein, also known as retinoid isomerohydrolase, is an enzyme of the vertebrate visual cycle and is encoded in humans by the RPE65 gene. *Voretigene neparvovec-rzyl* (Luxturna) is administered through subretinal injection, creating a well-supported bubble between the retina and the underlying epithelium, which corrects RPE65 deficiency in the retinal pigmented epithelium.

AAV2 became the first serotype to be clinically approved. It is used for the treatment of RPE65-related retinal dystrophy through gene replacement. The retinal pigment epithelium-specific 65 kDa protein, also known as retinoid isomerohydrolase, is an enzyme of the vertebrate visual cycle and is encoded in humans by the RPE65 gene. The AAV2 gene therapy product *voretigene neparvovec-rzyl* (Luxturna) has been approved for clinical use in 2017 (Figure 3.5).

*Eladocagene exuparvovec*, marketed as Upstaza, is a gene therapy used to treat severe aromatic L-amino acid decarboxylase (AADC) deficiency. This rare inherited condition affects the nervous system, leading to symptoms like developmental delays, weak muscle tone, and difficulty controlling limb movements. The therapy works by delivering a functional version of the AADC gene into nerve cells using an AAV2 enabling the production of the missing enzyme, which is crucial for dopamine synthesis - a neurotransmitter essential for movement control. It is administered for the treatment of patients aged 18 months and older with a clinical, molecular, and genetically confirmed diagnosis of AADC deficiency with a severe phenotype.

**AAV6** has been reported to mediate efficient transduction in lung airway epithelial cells and muscle cells. AAV6 is employed in various clinical applications and trials for cardiac disease, hemophilia, and liver diseases.

**AAV8**, in addition to AAV2 and AAV5, is the most widely used AAV serotype. AAV8 delivers genes very efficiently to the liver, skeletal muscle, and heart after intravenous administration. It is being used in several clinical trials.

**AAV9** displays a similar profile to AAV2, with higher efficiency. Quite importantly, AAV9 can, in a certain measure, cross the blood–brain barrier (BBB), thereby allowing gene delivery to neuronal tissue. An AAV9 has shown dramatic efficacy for the early treatment of spinal muscular atrophy in newborns, leading to the clinical approval in 2019 of *onasemnogene abeparvovec* (Zolgensma), a gene replacement therapy drug delivering the gene survival of motoneuron gene 1 (SMN1) to motor neuron cells, both in the spinal cord and in the brain. This surprising capacity of AAV9 to cross the BBB presumably occurs through transcytosis across endothelial cells from the brain capillaries, which are responsible for the BBB and are linked together by tight junctions. The brain penetration of AAV9 has been proven not only in animals but also in humans. Post-mortem tissue samples from two patients with SMA type 1 enrolled in a clinical trial demonstrated widespread biodistribution of *onasemnogene abeparvovec* vector genomes, mRNA transcripts, and SMN protein following intravenous administration. In both patients, *onasemnogene abeparvovec* crossed the BBB, and the SMN protein was expressed in neural tissues, such as the brain and spinal cord, in addition to peripheral tissues such as the heart, liver, and skeletal muscle.

**AAV5:** It is important to note that, in addition to its cellular tropism, the choice of a specific AAV might heavily depend on the absence of pre-existing immunity. Since human AAVs infect a large proportion of the population, the presence of neutralizing antibodies might severely affect the therapeutic outcome. Indeed, preexisting neutralizing antibodies against the AAV particles represent a major obstacle for AAV gene therapy development because neutralizing antibodies in the circulation are able to shield the receptor binding sites exposed on the capsid protein surface and thereby inactivate the viral vector. The preferential choice of AAV5 for two recently approved treatments, in which an intravenous AAV5 administration is performed, perfectly illustrates this preexisting immunity concern. These two gene drugs are as follows:

- *Etranacogene dezaparvovec* (Hemgenix), which has been approved in 2022 for hemophilia B through IV administration of an AAV5 for liver expression and secretion to the blood circulation of the clotting factor IX.
- *Valoctocogene roxaparvovec* (Roctavian), which has been approved in 2023 for hemophilia A through IV administration of an AAV5 for liver expression and secretion to the blood circulation of the clotting factor VIII.

In these two recent clinical applications, the AAV5 serotype was chosen due to its lower prevalence of preexisting immunity in the general population. This choice, however, was difficult since AAV5 is known to display low tropism and transduction efficiency in the liver. But AAV5 administration at moderate doses was found to be sufficient to restore blood's coagulation capacity safely. However, to extend the application of AAV5 for other liver-targeted diseases, more robust and specific gene delivery into hepatocytes (allowing less off-target tissue/organ transduction) might be needed.

AAVrh74 represents a typical example of a newly engineered AAV with enhanced tropism selectivity. The gene therapy treatment *delandistrogene moxeparvovec* (Elevidys) was approved in 2023 for Duchenne muscular dystrophy. It is delivered to treat ambulatory pediatric patients aged four through five years with Duchenne muscular dystrophy and a confirmed mutation in the DMD gene. The mode of administration is IV. The AAV serotype used is AAVrh74, which has several unique characteristics, as follows: (1) strong affinity and transduction efficiency for muscle tissue; (2) the prevalence of preexisting antibodies against AAVrh74 is generally lower compared to other serotypes such as AAV2 and AAV8, reducing the risk of neutralizing immune response; and (3) AAVrh74 has been designed to limit liver transduction (a "detargeting" action), which can be beneficial for therapies where liver transduction is undesired.

AAVrh74 has been derived from a rhesus monkey AAV serotype through capsid selection, based on the criteria for transduction in muscle cells. This was performed by screening various AAV serotypes to identify those with high transduction efficiency and specificity for muscle tissues (both skeletal and cardiac). In addition, a muscle-specific promoter, such as the muscle creatine kinase (MCK) promoter, is used for the transgene to ensure that the therapeutic gene is expressed specifically in muscle tissues. The AAVrh74 vector has been further optimized for improved transduction efficiency and a reduced immune response. This involved modifications to both the capsid and the genome.

## 3.3  Recombinant Viral Vectors Derived from Herpes Simplex 1

After initial infection and lytic multiplication at the body periphery, generally at oral or genital epithelial cells, the herpes simplex 1 (HSV-1) enters sensory nerve endings innervating the site of viral multiplication, and is retrogradely transported to the nucleus of sensory neurons. The mechanism of this retrograde transport along the axon occurs through the action of dynein, a motor protein, with the dynactin protein serving as a cofactor. Dynein moves along microtubules toward their minus end, which is typically oriented toward the cell body. This retrograde transport allows HSV-1 to establish latency or replicate. The HSV-1 genome replicates through a rolling circle mechanism, thus forming head-to-tail concatemers, a process which is used in recombinant vectors to package multiple copies of the gene of interest.

HSV-1 is an enveloped virus. Its genome is a linear dsDNA of 152 kb, encoding at least 80 gene products. The infectious virus particle contains an icosahedral core containing the viral DNA genome and core proteins. Around the core, 20 different proteins with structural and regulatory roles are found; they are surrounded by an external envelope containing different glycoproteins involved in various functions, including binding to cellular receptors and entry into the host cell. The HSV-1 primary cellular receptors include heparan sulfate proteoglycans, which are found on the surface of many cell types and facilitate the initial attachment of the virus, and Nectin-1, a member of the immunoglobulin superfamily. These key receptors allow HSV-1 entry, particularly into epithelial and neuronal cells. Another receptor is the protein Herpesvirus Entry Mediator (HVEM), a receptor present on cells of the immune system.

Three different classes of vectors can be derived from HSV-1: replication-competent attenuated vectors, replication-incompetent recombinant vectors, and defective helper-dependent vectors known as amplicons. The neurotrophic nature of HSV-1 makes it an attractive candidate for the transduction of neuronal cells; however, HSV-1-derived vectors have also proven valuable for other applications, such as an oncolytic viral vector (see Section 3.4) or for the treatment of skin diseases. Indeed HSV-1 viral vectors have already several clinical applications, including gene therapy, oncolytic virotherapy, and vaccines. These applications concern the vaccination against several viruses such as Ebola virus, foot-and-mouth disease virus, HIV. Cancer vaccines targeting cancer-associated antigens are also being developped using HSV-1 viral vectors.

The large packaging capacity of HSV-1 vectors makes them a preferred, sometimes unique, choice for delivering large genomes, as illustrated by the example of epidermolysis bullosa. Recessive dystrophic epidermolysis bullosa is a devastating rare genetic skin disease caused by loss-of-function mutations in the COL7A1 gene, encoding the collagen type VII alpha 1 chain. The protein collagen VII forms fibers which represent the structural component of the basement membrane between the epidermis and dermis, and it maintains epidermal adhesion to the deeper dermal layer. Epidermolysis bullosa results in severe symptoms such as painful blistering and fibrosis starting at birth, accompanied by scarring, susceptibility to infection, and a predisposition to skin cancer.

Various cell and gene strategies have been proposed for epidermolysis bullosa. Bone marrow transplantation with wild-type COL7A1 gene donors yields variable results and exhibits a high mortality rate. Alternatively, an autologous *ex vivo* approach consists of using a retroviral vector to stably introduce a functional COL7A1 gene into the patient's keratinocytes or using a self-inactivated SIN-lentiviral vector to stably transduce autologous fibroblasts. The size of the COL7A1 cDNA transgene needed for epidermolysis bullosa skin correction is about 9 kb. This exceeds the packaging capacity of most viral vectors, including AdVs, AAVs, and retro-/lentiviral vectors, which normally have a packaging capacity of about 8 kb. Thus, extensive modifications and optimizations of the retro-/lentiviral vectors were necessary to enable their delivery of functional COL7A1 cDNA. After *in vitro* expansion, the corrected cells were grafted onto the patient. This heavy procedure of *ex vivo* cell transduction and cellular expansion required grafting under general anesthesia for the keratinocyte approach and multiple local injections for the fibroblast approach, followed by postoperative graft immobilization. In addition, long-term clinical results were variable; they tended to decrease over time in some patients.

HSV-1 presents very attractive features for this particular disease. First, its large size capacity of about 40 kb allows us to package multiple copies of the COL7A1 gene. Second, it has developed robust molecular tools to evade the host's immune response. And third, it is a non-integrating vector, which suppresses the risk of insertional oncogenesis. This led to the development of the gene therapy drug *beremagene geperpavec* (B-VEC, VYJUVEK).

*Beremagene geperpavec* is a gene therapy based on topically applied, redosable, live, replication-defective HSV-1 used to deliver functional human COL7A1 genes in patients with both dominant and recessive dystrophic epidermolysis bullosa. *Beremagene geperpavec* contains two copies of the human COL7A1 cDNA and can transduce both keratinocytes and fibroblasts and restore functional COL7 protein. In 2023, *beremagene geperpavec* received its first approval in the US for treating wounds in patients older than six months of age with dystrophic epidermolysis bullosa with mutation(s) in the COL7A1 gene. This represents the first clinically approved topical gene therapy for skin diseases.

## 3.4 Oncolytic Viruses for Cancer Gene Therapy

Oncolytic viruses are constructed to specifically replicate only within cancer cells, without affecting normal cells, thus leading to selective cancer cell destruction. This destruction occurs either by the direct lytic effect of the virus or by inducing the body's innate and adaptive immune responses. Virus replication in cancer cells and its spread to adjacent tumor cells (a so-called "bystander effect") ensures the infection of a large number of tumor cells, hence achieving therapeutic efficacy through either stopping tumor growth or even leading to tumor elimination (Figure 3.6).

AdVs represent an intensively studied class of oncolytic viruses because of their high transduction efficacy, their amphotropic character allowing the infection of a broad range of tumor types, and their ability to induce a robust and strong immune-inflammatory response.

The construction of selectively or conditionally replicating recombinant AdVs mainly involves placing the E1A or E1B genes, which are essential for AdV replication, under the control of promoters selectively activated in tumors, as compared to normal tissue. Several promoters are

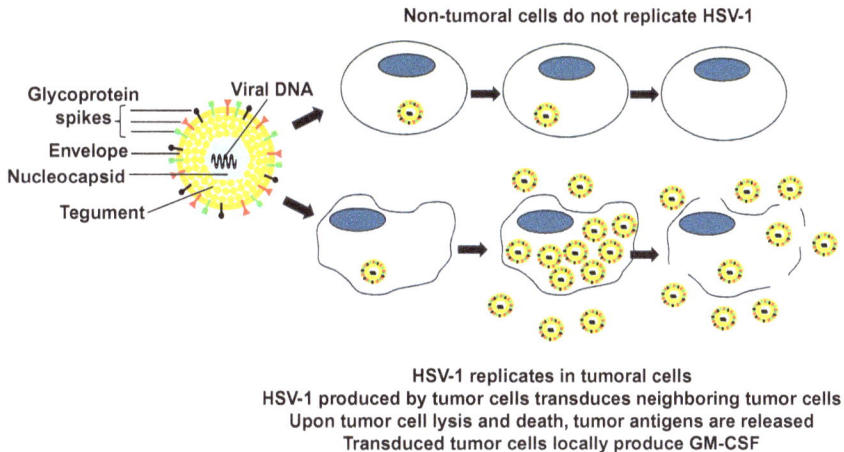

**Figure 3.6.** Schematic diagram of HSV-1 structure and the mechanism of action of an oncolytic HSV-1-derived recombinant vector. As in the case of *Talimogene laherparepvec* (see the following), the oncolytic HSV-1 has been engineered to secrete the immunostimulatory cytokine GM-CSF, thereby stimulating an anticancer immune response.

activated in most tumors, such as those of survivin, cyclooxygenase (COX-2), human telomerase reverse transcriptase hTERT, and other proteins involved in the stabilization, assembly, and function of the telomerase complex. Another strategy is to insert a hypoxia-response element into the promoter of essential viral proteins in order to take advantage of the fact that most solid tumors are hypoxic. Other oncolytic viruses contain essential viral genes under the dependence of a promoter specific to a given tumor type, such as prostate-specific antigen promoter, alpha-fetoprotein promoter activated in liver cancer, carcinoembryonic antigen promoter activated in epithelial cancer, and breast cancer specific promoter.

A large number of lytic viruses, other than AdVs, are being studied as oncolytic virus candidates. These include the types listed in Table 3.1.

In addition to their direct lytic effect on tumor cells, most oncolytic viruses incorporate immunostimulatory cytokine genes in order to enhance both the local innate immunity at the level of the tumor and the

**Table 3.1.**    Selected oncolytic viruses in clinical development.

| Oncolytic virus | Cancer clinical trials |
|---|---|
| Adenovirus | Bladder cancer, ovarian cancer, prostate cancer, head and neck cancer, sarcomas, NSCLC, glioblastoma |
| Coxsackie virus | Melanoma, breast cancer, prostate cancer |
| HSV-1 | Melanoma, breast cancer, head and neck cancer, pancreatic cancer |
| Measles virus | Ovarian cancer, glioblastoma, multiple myeloma |
| Newcastle disease virus | Glioblastoma |
| Parvovirus | Glioblastoma |
| Poliovirus | Glioblastoma |
| Poxvirus | Head and neck cancer, hepatocellular carcinoma, melanoma, colorectal cancer |
| Reovirus | non–small-cell lung cancer, ovarian cancer, melanoma, head and neck cancer |
| Seneca valley virus | Neuroblastoma, lung cancer |
| Vesicular stomatitis virus | Hepatocellular carcinoma |

*Source*: Reproduced from Kohlhapp and Kaufman (2015).

adaptive immune response against the tumor antigens released by the lytic process. Granulocyte macrophage colony-stimulating factor (GM-CSF) is the favored inflammatory cytokine for insertion into an oncolytic viral genome, although other inflammatory genes have also been proposed, such as IL-12, IL-18, CD40L, and 4-1BBL, which are expressed by an oncolytic virus either alone or jointly in order to enhance the ability of anti-tumor immune response.

*Talimogene laherparepvec* (T-VEC) is an oncolytic virus derived from HSV-1, which has been clinically approved for patients with melanoma. Research involving T-VEC has since been expanded to clinical trials involving patients with other cancers and combinations with other therapeutic agents. T-VEC has been genetically modified to specifically replicate within cancer cells, but not in normal cells. The HSV-1 neurovirulence gene has been deleted, preventing fever blister development. In addition, a viral HSV-1 gene that is responsible for evading immune response by blocking antigen presentation has been deleted, thus allowing the development of a robust immune response against infected tumor cells or non-infected tumor cells presenting a specific tumor antigen.

The mechanism of T-VEC selective replication in cancer cells is based on the fact that antiviral signaling pathways present in normal cells are generally disrupted in tumor cells, namely, the type I interferon and protein kinase R pathways. This allows preferential and selective HSV-1 replication within cancer cells. T-VEC also produces the immune response stimulatory protein, human GM-CSF, which helps to promote an immune response against cancer cells (Figure 3.6). These modifications, along with the unique environment of cancer cells, enable T-VEC to selectively target and destroy cancer cells while sparing normal cells.

Two other oncolytic viruses have been approved in one or a few countries for the treatment of advanced cancer. Rigvir is an oncolytic virus derived from the ECHO-7 strain of enterovirus, which has been approved in Latvia for the treatment of melanoma, and Oncorine (H101 AdV) is a genetically modified AdV approved in China for the treatment of head and neck cancer. It is expected that many more oncolytic viruses will find their way to clinical use in the future.

# Bibliography

## *Adenoviral vectors*

Sayedahmed EE, Kumari R, Mittal SK. Current use of adenovirus vectors and their production methods. *Methods Mol Biol.* 2019;1937:155–175. doi: 10.1007/978-1-4939-9065-8_9.

Zhang H, Wang H, An Y, Chen Z. Construction and application of adenoviral vectors. *Mol Ther Nucleic Acids.* 2023 Sep;34:102027. doi: 10.1016/j.omtn.2023.09.004.

## *Adeno-associated viral vectors*

Blair H. Onasemnogene abeparvovec: a review in spinal muscular atrophy. *CNS Drugs.* 2022;36:995–1005. doi.org/10.1007/s40263-022-00941-1.

Dhillon S. Beremagene geperpavec: first approval. *Drugs.* 2023 Aug;83(12): 1131–1135. doi: 10.1007/s40265-023-01921-5.

Hoffman JA, Denton N, Sims JJ, Meggersee R, Zhang Z, Olagbegi K, Wilson JM. Modulation of AAV9 galactose binding yields novel gene therapy vectors and predicts cross-species differences in glycan avidity. *Hum Gene Ther.* 2024 Sep;35(17–18):734–753. doi: 10.1089/hum.2024.050.

Kohlhapp FJ, Kaufman HL. Molecular pathways: mechanism of action for talimogene laherparepvec, a new oncolytic virus immunotherapy. *Clin Cancer Res.* 2016 Mar;22(5):1048–1054. doi: 10.1158/1078-0432.CCR-15-2667.

Meyer NL, Chapman MS. Adeno-associated virus (AAV) cell entry: structural insights. *Trends Microbiol.* 2022 May;30(5):432–451. doi: 10.1016/j.tim.2021.09.005.

Ronzitti G, Gross DA, Mingozzi F. Human immune responses to adeno-associated virus (AAV) vectors. *Front Immunol.* 2020 Apr;11:670. doi: 10.3389/fimmu.2020.00670.

Shchaslyvyi AY, Antonenko SV, Tesliuk MG, Telegeev GD. Current state of human gene therapy: approved products and vectors. *Pharmaceuticals.* 2023 Oct;16(10):1416. doi: 10.3390/ph16101416.

Wang Y, Yang C, Hu H, Chen C, Yan M, Ling F, Wang KC, Wang X, *et al.* Directed evolution of adeno-associated virus 5 capsid enables specific liver tropism. *Mol Ther Nucleic Acids.* 2022 Mar;28:293–306. doi: 10.1016/j.omtn.2022.03.017.

## *Recombinant viral vectors derived from herpes simplex 1*

Gurevich I, Agarwal P, Zhang P, Dolorito JA, Oliver S, Liu H, Reitze N, Sarma N, *et al. In vivo* topical gene therapy for recessive dystrophic epidermolysis bullosa: a phase 1 and 2 trial. *Nat Med.* 2022 Apr;28(4):780–788. doi: 10.1038/s41591-022-01737-y.

Marconi P, Argnani R, Epstein AL, Manservigi R. HSV as a vector in vaccine development and gene therapy. *Adv Exp Med Biol.* 2009;655:118–144. doi: 10.1007/978-1-4419-1132-2_10.

## *Oncolytic viruses for cancer gene therapy*

Shalhout SZ, Miller DM, Emerick KS, Kaufman HL. Therapy with oncolytic viruses: progress and challenges. *Nat Rev Clin Oncol.* 2023 Mar;20(3): 160–177. doi: 10.1038/s41571-022-00719-w.

# Chapter 4

# Integrative Vectors Derived from Retroviruses and Lentiviruses

## 4.1 Integrative Viral Vectors Derived from Retroviruses and Lentiviruses

Retroviruses are a large family of RNA viruses which insert their retrotranscribed genome into host cells. Retroviruses have been classified into several groups based on their genetic structure and the diseases they cause. Among this large family, one can distinguish oncoretroviruses, which are associated with cancer and are subdivided into alpha, beta, gamma, delta, and epsilon subgroups, lentiviruses and spumaviruses. Lentiviruses comprise the human immunodeficiency virus (HIV), which is the causative agent of acquired immunodeficiency syndrome (AIDS). Note that oncoretroviruses are often indifferently named just "retroviruses" in most of the literature and also in the present textbook.

For gene therapy applications, two retro-/lentiviruses have been primarily used and are now available in clinics: (1) the recombinant, non-infective, replication-deficient gamma-oncoretrovirus derived from the Moloney murine leukemia virus (MoMuLV) and (2) the HIV-1-derived lentivirus. There are several key differences between these two types of vectors, which point to a preferential use of HIV-1-derived lentivirus. First, oncoretroviruses can only integrate their retrotranscribed genetic payload into the chromosomes of dividing mitotic cells, while lentivirus-derived vectors can perform this genome integration also in resting non-dividing cells. This represents a decisive advantage for lentiviruses in certain applications, such as transducing neurons or non-dividing T-lymphocytes. Second, lentiviral vectors are presently considered safer than gamma-oncoretroviral vectors in terms of their semi-random integration pattern, since lentiviral gene integration does not preferentially occur in the vicinity of actively transcribed genes, in contrast to gamma-oncoretroviruses. Third, while some oncoretroviruses, such as murine retroviruses, are inactivated by human complement, this is not the case for HIV-1-derived lentiviral vectors, making them more easily usable *in vivo*. And fourth, the MoMuLV induces a strong immune response, such as by activating cytolytic T lymphocytes which are specific for both viral and tumor-associated antigens, while HIV-1 vectors exhibit low immunogenicity.

Oncoretroviruses and lentiviruses are enveloped viruses. Their genome consists of two copies of positive-sense single-stranded RNA (ssRNA) molecules of 8.3 kb in size for the wild-type oncoretroviruses and 9.7 kb for the wild-type HIV-1. For both oncoretroviruses and lentiviruses, the ssRNA is packaged into a core nucleocapsid which contains a reverse transcriptase (*pol* gene) responsible for generating the retrotranscribed double-stranded DNA (dsDNA) viral genome, an integrase responsible for integration into the host cell genome, and a protease which is responsible for the maturation of the GAG and POL proteins.

The nucleocapsid core of gamma-oncoretrovirus and lentivirus contains several key proteins that are essential for its structure and function. These include the nucleocapsid NC protein, which packages and coats the retroviral RNA genome and is important for RNA protection, the core protein CA, and the matrix M protein, which is associated with the inner leaflet of the viral membrane and contributes to the assembly and stability of the viral particle.

Another important protein is glycosaminoglycan GAG, which is essential for several key functions in the viral replication cycle, such as viral assembly, intracellular transport to the cell membrane of viral components, the budding process where new viral particles are released from the host cell, gene expression regulation, and interaction with the host proteins. The glycosaminoglycan GAG polyprotein encodes matrix (MA), capsid (CA), and nucleocapsid (NC).

The external lipid membranes of oncoretro-/lentiviruses contain proteins encoded by the *env* gene. These are mainly glycoproteins. In HIV-1 for instance, the main envelope proteins are gp120, the glycoprotein responsible for binding to the CD4 receptor on host cells, and gp41, a glycoprotein embedded in the viral envelope which facilitates the fusion of the viral membrane with the host cell membrane. Together, gp120 and gp41 form a complex that allows HIV-1 to enter and infect host cells.

The production of a recombinant lentiviral vector is displayed in Figure 4.1. The therapeutic expression cassette is flanked in 5' by a long terminal repeat (LTR) and an encapsidation psi ($\psi$) sequence and in 3' by the second LTR. The $\psi$ sequence plays an essential role in the recognition and packaging of viral RNA in the nucleocapsid. In the context of gene therapy, the $\psi$ sequence ensures that the therapeutic expression cassette is selectively included in the viral particles, enabling their delivery to target cells, with the exclusion of lentiviral genes which are not adjacent to a $\psi$ sequence.

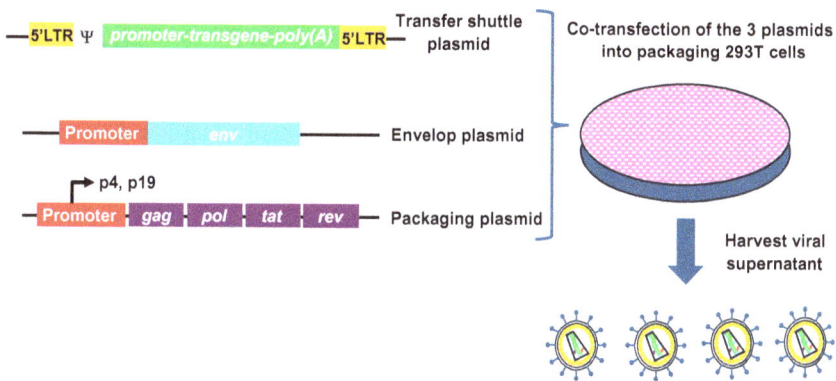

**Figure 4.1.** Production of a recombinant lentiviral vector through multiple plasmid co-transfection. *env*: envelope gene, *gag*: gene of the protein core of the virus, *pol*: gene of the reverse transcriptase which produces retrotranscribed dsDNA, *tat*: trans-activator of transcription, *rev*: regulator of the virion gene. In contrast to AdV or AAV vectors, for which the lysis of packaging cells is required for vector production, the recombinant oncoretro- and lentiviruses are collected in the supernatant of the cultured cells because they need to bud from the packaging cells as enveloped viruses.

The LTRs facilitate the integration of the viral genome into the host cell's DNA, which is essential for stable gene expression. In addition, LTRs contain promoter and enhancer elements that regulate the transcription of the viral genome. The 5' LTR acts as a promoter for the transcription of the viral RNA, while the 3' LTR contains signals for the polyadenylation and termination of transcription. In some lentiviral vectors, the 3' LTR is modified to create a "self-inactivating" (SIN) vector. This modification reduces the risk of activating oncogenes in the genome of the patient's cells, thereby enhancing the safety of the vector (see Section 4.3).

The envelope gene (*env*) might not correspond to the endogenous wild-type oncoretro- or lentiviral envelope genes since, in order to broaden vector tropism, it is often replaced by the vesicular stomatitis virus glycoprotein envelope gene (*vsv-g*). The vector is then designated as "pseudotyped". The VSV-G surface protein is commonly used for pseudotyping oncoretroviral and lentiviral vectors due to several key advantages, as follows: (i) VSV-G can bind to LDL receptor family members, allowing the virus to infect a wide range of cell types from various species, including rodent and human cells; (ii) VSV-G pseudotyped vectors exhibit increased stability, which is beneficial for maintaining the integrity of the viral particles during storage and handling; (iii) and finally, VSV-G pseudotyped vectors tend to have higher infectious titers, meaning they can deliver their genetic payload more efficiently. However, it is worth noting that VSV-G can be cytotoxic to producer cells. While this issue has been mitigated by using tetracycline-regulated promoters, the development of stable producer cell lines for lentivectors pseudotyped with VSV-G still represents a challenge, owing to the cytotoxicity associated with this envelope, which is not the case with other vector envelopes.

In addition to genes encoding the envelope *env*, glycosaminoglycan (*gag*) and reverse transcriptase (*pol*) genes, the packaging cells are co-transfected with the trans-activator of transcription (*tat*) and regulator of virion (*rev*) genes. These are crucial components of the lentiviral system, particularly in the context of HIV-1. The *tat* gene encodes a protein that significantly enhances the efficiency of viral transcription by binding to a region of the viral RNA called the trans-activation response (TAR) element, which is located at the 5' end of all nascent viral transcripts. This interaction recruits cellular factors that increase the processivity of RNA polymerase II, thereby boosting the transcription of viral genes. The *rev* gene encodes a protein that is essential for the export of unspliced and singly spliced viral RNAs from the nucleus to the cytoplasm. The REV protein binds to a specific RNA sequence, known as the Rev response element (RRE), present in these RNAs. This binding facilitates their transport out of the nucleus, allowing them to be translated into viral proteins or packaged into new virions.

Oncoretroviral and lentiviral entry into host cells is schematized in Figure 4.2. Briefly, the successive entry steps are as follows, by taking HIV-1 lentivirus as an example:

(1) Binding to specific cell surface receptors on the host cell. First, HIV-1 gp120 binds to CD4, then to the coreceptors CXCR4 and CCR5.

(2) The viral envelope fuses with the host cell membrane, allowing the viral core to be delivered to the cytoplasm. This fusion step fundamentally differs from that of adenovirus or AAV, which occurs through endosome internalization via coated pits and fusion promoted

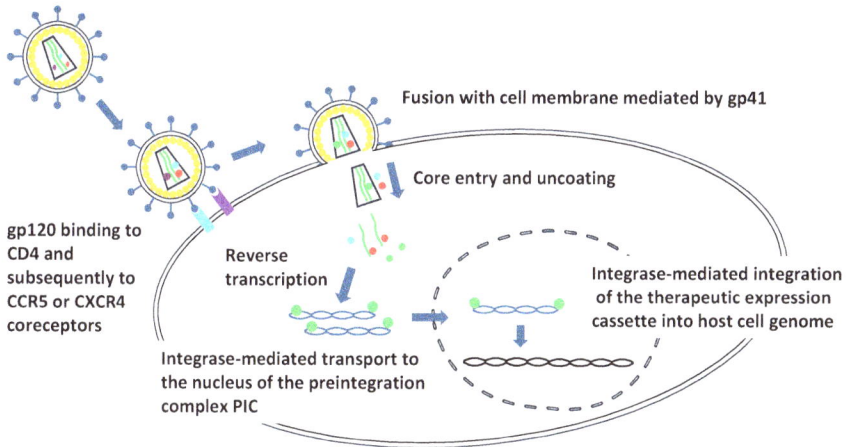

**Figure 4.2.** Lentiviral entry into host cells. The matrix proteins are represented as yellow circles. The core is schematized as a black trapezoid. Key proteins involved in the entry and integration include the protease (violet circle), the reverse transcriptase (red circle), and the integrase (green circle).

by endosomal acidification. For oncoretro- and lentiviruses, no acidi-fication-dependent structural change of fusion proteins is necessary since the fusion step involves the host cell receptor as a trigger for the gp41 envelope protein conformational change, which drives membrane fusion.

(3) Core uncoating in the cytoplasm leads to viral RNA reverse transcription into dsDNA by the enzyme reverse transcriptase. This step differs from the case of AAV, for which capsid uncoating occurs in the nucleus.

(4) For oncoretroviruses, retroviral DNA integration mediated by the integrase protein occurs during the mitotic state, while for lentiviruses, the viral genome is transported through the nuclear pores and further integrated into the host chromosomes.

## 4.2 Early Clinical Successes

Oncoretro- and lentiviruses are necessary when stable transgene expression is required in actively dividing cells, such as stem cells or cytotoxic T lymphocytes, because only chromosomal integration ensures stable transgene expression, while episomal transgenes are lost upon cell division. Several research studies have reported *in vivo* use of HIV-1-derived vectors. However, in actual clinical settings, this integration property has been only used in *ex vivo* gene therapy protocols (Figure 4.3).

One of the first success of gene therapy has concerned the treatment of Severe Combined Immunodeficiency (SCID) using the Moloney murine leukemia gamma-oncoretroviral vector, which was published in 2000 by French and Italian teams. SCID is a rare, life-threatening primary immunodeficiency disorder characterized by the combined absence of T cell and B cell functions. Patients with SCID have a severely compromised immune system, making them extremely vulnerable to infections; thus, they require living in a completely germ-free, controlled environment — hence the term "bubble babies", referring to SCID children, many of whom are forced to live in sterile environments, often referred to as "bubbles", to protect them from germs.

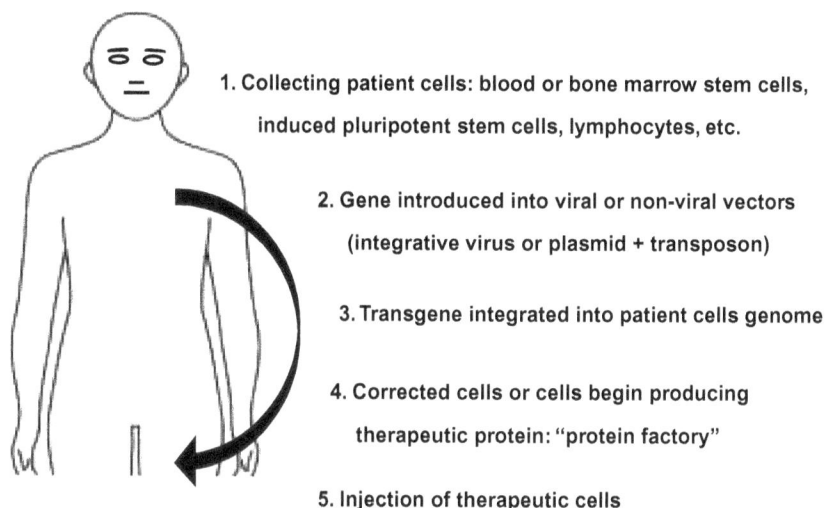

1. Collecting patient cells: blood or bone marrow stem cells, induced pluripotent stem cells, lymphocytes, etc.

2. Gene introduced into viral or non-viral vectors (integrative virus or plasmid + transposon)

3. Transgene integrated into patient cells genome

4. Corrected cells or cells begin producing therapeutic protein: "protein factory"

5. Injection of therapeutic cells

**Figure 4.3.**   *Ex vivo* gene therapy process. In this autologous protocol, patient cells are collected and stably transduced using either oncoretroviral or lentiviral vectors. An alternative strategy, leading also to stable chromosomal integration by using transposons, is described in Chapter 3.

The X-linked subtype of SCID disease (X-SCID) is the most common form and is caused by mutations in the *il2r*γ gene located on the X chromosome, a gene which encodes the interleukin-2 receptor common gamma chain (γc) of the receptor for the activation cytokine interleukin-2 (IL-2) on immune cells. The defective part of the lymphocyte receptor is the gamma chain, which is a common component of lymphocyte receptors for several types of cytokines, including IL-2. Thus, it is a critical component for mobilizing the body's defenses against infection.

Figure 4.4 displays the *ex vivo* gene therapy strategy used to restore a functional IL-2 receptor on lymphocytes in the first historical X-SCID clinical trial. The viral vector used was a MoMuLV oncoretroviral vector. The *il2r*γc DNA was flanked by the two LTRs of the wild-type oncoretrovirus and the encapsidation ψ sequence. In the initial clinical protocol, CD 34+ hematopoietic stem/progenitor cells (HSPCs) were collected from the patient, cultured, and briefly stimulated to start the cell division process before transduction. About one million cells were readministered to the patient, which allowed for the reconstitution of a fully competent

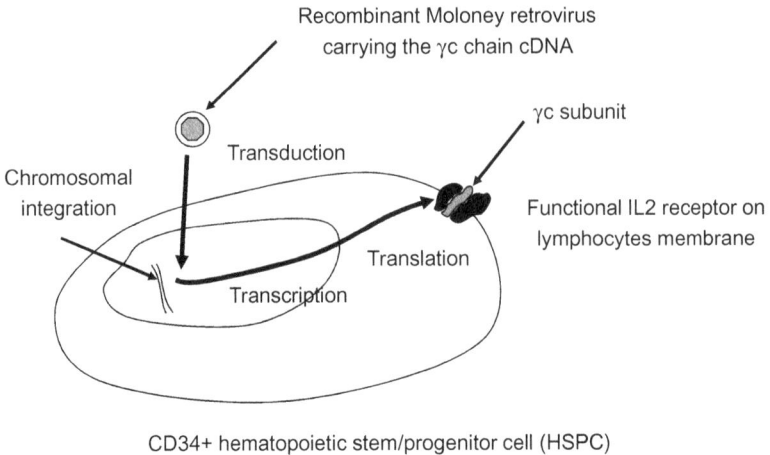

**Figure 4.4.** Gene therapy strategy used for restoring a functional IL-2 receptor on lymphocytes in the first X-SCID clinical trial. In a typical protocol, HSPCs are pre-stimulated by culture with cytokines such as stem cell factor (SCF), Flt-3 ligand, and thrombopoietin (TPO) to stimulate their proliferation and maintain their stem cell properties. The pre-stimulated HSPCs are then transduced with a oncoretro- or lentiviral vector carrying the therapeutic gene. This step is crucial for introducing the corrective gene into the HSPCs. After transduction, the cells are further cultured with cytokines to ensure their viability and expansion before being infused back into the patient. These steps help ensure that the HSPCs are effectively modified and can be engrafted onto the patient's bone marrow to produce functional immune cells.

immunological repertoire and the restoration of efficient immune protection in the patient.

Another form of SCID, ADA-SCID, is caused by the deficiency of the enzyme adenosine deaminase, which is produced by a gene on chromosome 20. Adenosine deaminase is involved in the metabolism of purines, which are essential building blocks of DNA and RNA. Its primary role is to catalyze the conversion of adenosine to inosine, a crucial step in the breakdown of adenosine from food and the turnover of nucleic acids in tissues. In humans, ADA is particularly important for the development and maintenance of the immune system. Gene therapy of ADA-SCID was performed for the first time in Italy using, as with X-linked SCID, a Moloney murine leukemia gamma-oncoretroviral vector.

## 4.3 Genotoxic Insertional Oncogenesis and Self-Inactivated Retro-/Lentiviral Vectors

Initially, this X-linked SCID gene therapy showed promising results, with some children experiencing significant improvements. However, some participants in the clinical trial later developed leukemia. Most, but not all, were cured. It was rapidly discovered that these leukemias were caused by the reactivation of the LMO2 oncogene due to the strong promoter/enhancer effects of the LTRs.

LMO2 is an oncogene that plays a crucial role in the early development of the hematopoietic system. It is a transcriptional regulator involved in the formation of a complex that controls gene expression necessary for blood cell development. It is repressed during late developmental stages. However, when LMO2 is abnormally reactivated, it can lead to the development of T-cell acute lymphoblastic leukemia (T-ALL).

In the case of the X-linked SCID trial, it was shown that acute lymphoblastic leukemia cells derived from a single clonal insertion near the LMO2 gene, leading to its unintended distant activation by the LTR. The probability of such an event occurring was quite high since about one million T-cells had been randomly transduced by the retroviral vector.

Similarly, despite the fact that the ADA-SCID gamma-retroviral gene therapy received clinical approval in 2016 under the name of Strimvelis (CD34+ hematopoietic stem/progenitor cell (HSPC) transduced *ex vivo* with the ADA gene under the control of the viral LTR promoter/enhancer), several leukemias have been described for ADA-SCID patients treated with this gene therapy. This was also the case for patients treated with retroviral gene therapy for other immune deficiencies, such as chronic granulomatous disease (CGD) and Wiskott–Aldrich syndrome (WAS).

This unwanted severe LTR-related genotoxic side effect, coined as "insertional oncogenesis", considerably slowed down the development of the use of retro-/lentiviral vectors until this bottleneck was resolved by the introduction of self-inactivated (SIN) vectors. Both SIN oncoretroviral and lentiviral vectors have been developed based on the elucidation of the LTR's internal structure and function.

As an illustration, the HIV-1 LTRs, which play a significant role in the virus' replication and integration into the host genome, are divided into three main regions: U3, R, and U5. Region U3 (Unique 3') is located at the 3' end of each LTR and contains important regulatory elements, including enhancers and promoters that are essential for the initiation of viral transcription. Region R (Repeat) is a short sequence found in both the 5' and 3' LTRs which plays a role in the reverse transcription process and contains the transcription start site. Region U5 (Unique 5') is located at the 5' end of each LTR and contains sequences necessary for the integration of viral DNA into the host genome. These regions work together to ensure the proper transcription, replication, and integration of the HIV-1 virus.

An example of a SIN-lentivirus genome construct used in a clinical trial is presented in Figure 4.5. Briefly, a SIN-lentiviral vector is produced as replication-defective viral particles in which the RNA genome contains a so-called SIN 3LTR, which upon reverse transcription into a linear dsDNA genome gives rise to an U3-deleted LTR, devoid of enhancer and promoter capacities. The U3 LTRs must maintain a minimum of an 18 bp long HIV-1 sequence necessary for integration, as well as the R and U5 regions containing the vector polyadenylation sequence. The genome maintains the cis-acting viral sequences necessary for encapsidation, reverse transcription, and integration into the host cell genome but lacks all

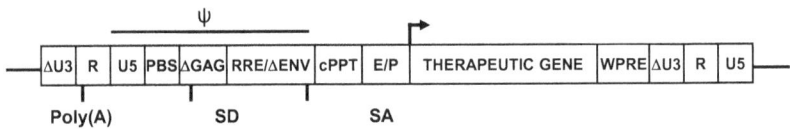

**Figure 4.5.** A prototype, third-generation LV provirus, featuring a disabling (SIN) deletion of the enhancer/promoter sequences in the U3 region of the LTR up to position -18 from the viral transcription start site. The poly(A) signal-containing R and the U5 regions of the LTR are retained. PBS, primer binding site; ΔGAG, deleted, non-coding portion of the GAG gene containing the D1 major HIV-1 splice donor (SD) site (CTG/GTGAGTAC); RRE, Rev responsive element; ΔENV, deleted portion of the ENV gene containing the A7 HIV-1 splice acceptor (SA) site (TCGTTTCAG/A); cPPT, central polypurine tract; E/P, enhancer/promoter component of the expression cassette (the arrow represents the transcription start site); WPRE, woodchuck hepatitis virus post-transcriptional regulatory element; ψ, extended packaging signal.

*Source*: Adapted from Poletti and Mavilio (2021).

other viral regulatory elements and genes, which are replaced by the transgene cargo. The necessarily maintained sequences are the packaging signal ($\psi$), the primer binding site (PBS), and the polypurine tract (PPT), which is required for reverse transcription. In addition, the recombinant lentiviral vector also contains the major HIV-1 intron with donor and acceptor splice sites and the Rev responsive element (RRE) required for the Rev-mediated nuclear export of the unspliced, full genomic transcript.

The SIN-lentiviral vectors have been approved for clinical use in 2023 for the treatment of hemoglobinopathies, such as $\beta$-thalassemia and sickle cell disease. These therapies use lentiviral vectors to insert functional copies of the $\beta$-globin gene into the patient's hematopoietic stem cells, allowing for the production of functional hemoglobin (see Section 4.4). Other strategies are envisioned for hemoglobinopathies, with some of them using genome editing through the use of lentiviral vector-mediated transduction (Chapter 9).

## 4.4 Extension of Retro-/Lentiviral Clinical Use

Gamma-oncoretroviral vectors, as well as now-predominantly HIV-1-derived lentiviral vectors, have become current clinical practice in immuno-oncology for the cell/gene therapy of cancer using CAR-T cells (Chapter 8). They are also used to treat monogenic diseases, such as X-linked severe combined immunodeficiency (X-SCID), adenosine deaminase severe combined immunodeficiency (ADA-SCID), and chronic granulomatous disease (CGD).

A lentiviral vector has been used in humans for cerebral adrenoleuko-dystrophy (CALD), a rare X-linked genetic disorder that affects the brain and results from the accumulation of very long-chain fatty acids (VLCFAs) in the central nervous system. Adrenoleukodystrophy, a neurological disorder, is caused by mutations in the ABCD1 gene (also called ALD, or ATP-binding cassette, sub-family D, member 1). The ABCD1 gene encodes the adrenoleukodystrophy protein (ALDP), which is located in the membrane of peroxisomes and is involved in the transport of VLCFAs from the cytosol to the peroxisome interior, where VLCFAs are degraded by $\beta$-oxidative catabolism. Non-functional ALDP leads to the accumulation of VLCFAs in the brain and adrenal cortex, with severe detrimental effects on the nervous system and adrenal glands.

Before the introduction of gene therapy, the treatment of adrenoleukodystrophy was based on allogenic stem cell transplantation from a matching donor, with the risk of graft-versus-host disease. The gene therapy protocol involves collecting autologous CD34+ hematopoietic stem cells from the patient and transduction with a lentiviral vector carrying a functional copy of the ABCD1 gene. The genetically modified HSCs are then reinfused back into the patient, engraft in the bone marrow, and begin producing cells that express the functional ABCD1 protein. As a result, the accumulation of VLCFAs in the brain and other tissues is reduced, halting the progression of the disease and preventing further neurological damage. The gene therapy biologics is called *elivaldogene autotemcel* (eli-cel), marketed as Skysona.

*Atidarsagene autotemcel*, marketed as Libmeldy, is a gene therapy used to treat metachromatic leukodystrophy (MLD). MLD is a rare genetic disorder caused by mutations in the ARSA gene, leading to a deficiency of the enzyme arylsulfatase A. This deficiency results in the accumulation of sulfatides, which damage the protective myelin sheath around nerve cells, causing progressive neurological decline. The patient's hematopoietic stem cells are collected, genetically engineered to include a functional copy of the ARSA gene using a lentiviral vector, and then infused back into the patient. This allows the body to produce the missing enzyme, helping to slow or halt the progression of the disease. This therapy is typically used for children with early-onset forms of MLD, before significant symptoms develop. It is administered as a one-time intravenous infusion in specialized medical centers.

$\beta$-globin gene disorders are the most prevalent inherited diseases worldwide and result from abnormal $\beta$-globin synthesis or structure. The majority of these diseases comprises beta-thalassemia and sickle cell anemia.

Beta-thalassemia is caused by mutations or deletions in the *beta-globin* ($\beta$-globin) gene on chromosome 11. These genetic defects lead to reduced (beta+) or absent (beta0) synthesis of the beta chains of hemoglobin (Hb), resulting in an excess of alpha-globin chains. These unmatched alpha-globin chains precipitate within erythroid precursors in the bone marrow, damaging their membranes and leading to their accelerated apoptosis, premature destruction, and anemia. Severe anemia requires regular blood transfusions.

Sickle cell anemia is also caused by a mutation in the beta-globin subunit of hemoglobin. This mutation results in the substitution of valine for glutamic acid at the sixth position of the $\beta$-globin chain, leading to the production of an abnormal form of hemoglobin called hemoglobin S (HbS). Under low oxygen conditions, HbS molecules polymerize, forming long, rigid rods within red blood cells, causing them to become rigid, sticky, and sickle-shaped. The sickle-shaped cells can block blood flow in small blood vessels, leading to pain and tissue damage. In addition, sickle-shaped red blood cells (erythrocytes) are more fragile and prone to breaking apart. While normal erythrocytes live for about 120 days, sickle erythrocytes typically last only 10–20 days. This rapid breakdown leads to a shortage of red blood cells, causing chronic anemia and its associated complications.

Novel therapeutic approaches have been developed in an effort to move beyond palliative management in both beta-thalassemia and sickle cell anemia. Gene therapy, through the *ex vivo* lentiviral transfer of a therapeutic $\beta$-globin gene derivative ($\beta$AT87Q-globin) to hematopoietic stem cells, driven by cis-regulatory elements that confer high, erythroid-specific expression, has been evaluated in human clinical trials for more than a decade. In these clinical trials, $\beta$AT87Q-globin was used both as a strong inhibitor of HbS polymerization, the pathologic process responsible for sickle cell anemia, and as a biomarker to identify potential correction of beta-thalassemia. Proof of principle of efficacy and safety has been obtained in multiple patients. These two major indications concerning hemoglobinopathies and using SIN-lentiviral vectors have been clinically approved in 2023.

*Betibeglogene Autotemcel* (Zynteglo) is indicated for the treatment of patients aged 12 years and older with transfusion-dependent $\beta$-thalassemia who do not have a $\beta0/\beta0$ genotype and for whom HSC transplantation is appropriate but a human leukocyte antigen (HLA)-matched related HSC donor is not available. *Betibeglogene Autotemcel* works by adding functional copies of a modified $\beta$-globin gene ($\beta$A-T87Q-globin) to the patient's own hematopoietic stem cells (HSCs), *ex vivo*, via transduction of autologous CD34+ cells with a lentiviral vector (BB305 LVV). As for the adrenoleukodystrophy protocol, after infusion, the transduced CD34+ HSCs engraft in the bone marrow and differentiate to produce red blood cells containing biologically active $\beta$A-T87Q-globin. This modified $\beta$-globin pairs with $\alpha$-globin to produce functional hemoglobin (HbA T87Q), which helps correct the $\alpha/\beta$-globin imbalance and enables the production of functional hemoglobin, reducing the need for regular red blood cell transfusions.

*Lovotibeglogene Autotemcel* (LentiGlobin) is indicated for the treatment of patients aged 12 years and older with sickle cell disease who have a history of vaso-occlusive events. LentiGlobin involves, using the same protocol as for *Betibeglogene Autotemcel,* the autologous transplantation of hematopoietic stem and progenitor cells transduced with a lentiviral vector encoding a modified $\beta$-globin gene ($\beta$A-T87Q-globin). The modified $\beta$-globin gene helps produce hemoglobins with a similar oxygen-binding capacity as the wild-type hemoglobin and inhibits HbS polymerization, thus limiting the sickling of red blood cells.

## Bibliography

Dunbar CE. A plethora of gene therapies for hemoglobinopathies. *Nat Med.* 2021 Feb;27(2):202–204. doi: 10.1038/s41591-021-01235-7.

Fischer A. Gene therapy for inborn errors of immunity: past, present and future. *Nat Rev Immunol.* 2023 Jun;23(6):397–408. doi: 10.1038/s41577-022-00800-6.

Ghosh S, Brown AM, Jenkins C, Campbell K. Viral vector systems for gene therapy: a comprehensive literature review of progress and biosafety challenges. *Appl Biosaf.* 2020 Mar;25(1):7–18. doi: 10.1177/1535676019899502.

Martínez-Molina E, Chocarro-Wrona C, Martínez-Moreno D, Marchal JA, Boulaiz H. Large-scale production of lentiviral vectors: current perspectives and challenges. *Pharmaceutics*. 2020 Nov;12(11):1051. doi: 10.3390/pharmaceutics12111051.

Milani M, Canepari C, Liu T, Biffi M, Russo F, Plati T, Curto R, Patarroyo-White S, *et al*. Liver-directed lentiviral gene therapy corrects hemophilia A mice and achieves normal-range factor VIII activity in non-human primates. *Nat Commun*. 2022 May;13(1):2454. doi: 10.1038/s41467-022-30102-3.

Negre O, Eggimann AV, Beuzard Y, Ribeil JA, Bourget P, Borwornpinyo S, Hongeng S, Hacein-Bey S. Gene therapy of the $\beta$-hemoglobinopathies by lentiviral transfer of the $\beta$(A(T87Q))-globin gene. *Hum Gene Ther*. 2016 Feb;27(2):148–65. doi: 10.1089/hum.2016.007.

Poletti V, Mavilio F. Designing lentiviral vectors for gene therapy of genetic diseases. *Viruses*. 2021 Aug;13(8):1526. doi: 10.3390/v13081526.

# Chapter 5

# Non-Viral Gene Expression Vectors

## 5.1 Non-Viral DNA Expressing Vectors: Plasmids

Plasmids represent a widespread non-viral expression vector for gene therapy. Plasmids are double-stranded, circular DNA produced in a bacterial host at a high copy number, depending on the strength of their replication origin and their size. Up to 1,000 copies per bacterium can be obtained in the most efficiently engineered bacterial host. The most commonly used bacterial host for plasmid production is *Escherichia coli* (*E. coli*), which has multiple advantages. *E. coli* can produce high yields of plasmid DNA, making it an efficient host for plasmid production. *E. coli* is easy to grow and can be cultivated in large-scale bioreactors. *E. coli* is well studied and can be genetically manipulated to enhance plasmid production. Finally, *E. coli* K-12 strains are non-pathogenic and are widely accepted by regulatory agencies as gene therapy vectors.

Plasmid size is highly variable, ranging from 1.5 kilobase (kb) pairs up to 120 kb. In the gene therapy context, plasmids contain a eukaryotic expression cassette, which leads to the production of the desired mRNA or protein in target cells. This involves the cellular and nuclear delivery of the plasmid, a process called transfection, which is carried out on animal or human cells for the expression of therapeutic proteins or mRNA within the patient's cells. Alternatively, plasmids are also extensively used for the production of recombinant viral gene therapy vectors in eukaryotic cells (Chapters 2–4).

A typical gene therapy plasmid is displayed in Figure 5.1. The transcription unit, also called a transgene expression cassette or therapeutic expression cassette, comprises a eukaryotic promoter, the gene of interest (GOI), and the poly(A) untranslated region. The GOI is either a single therapeutic cDNA or a group of viral genes for the production of recombinant viral vectors.

In some cases, two or more cDNA sequences separated by an internal ribosomal entry site (IRES), are inserted into the plasmid. An IRES is a specific RNA sequence that allows for the initiation of translation in a cap-independent manner, thus allowing the expression of multiple genes from a single mRNA transcript. This means that the ribosome can translate the mRNA sequence into protein without the need for the typical 5' cap structure that usually initiates this process. IRES elements enable the

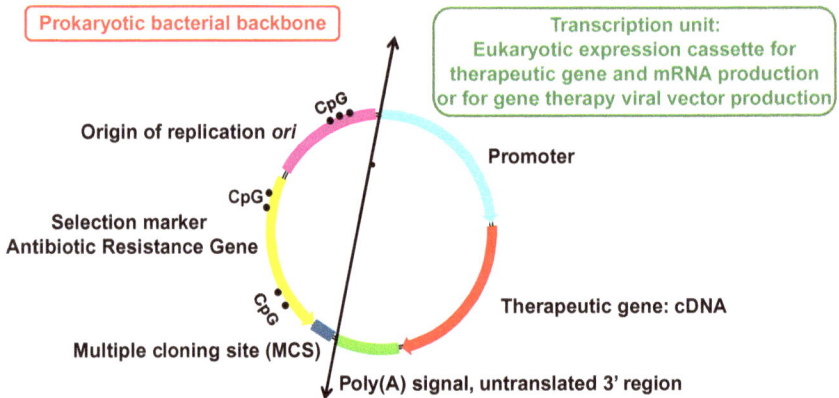

**Figure 5.1.** Structure of a plasmid vector. On the right side of the arrow, the transcription unit, also called the therapeutic expression cassette, comprises a eukaryotic promoter, the therapeutic cDNA, and the poly(A) untranslated region. On the left side of the arrow, the plasmid bacterial backbone contains a bacterial origin of replication and a selection marker. Prokaryotic sequences contain CpG motifs, which have immune-inflammatory properties and activate innate immune responses via Toll-like receptors. The multiple cloning site contains a high number of nucleic acid restriction sites, allowing for easy insertion of multiple transcription units, each containing diverse genes of interest (GOIs).

ribosome to bind directly to the mRNA and begin translation. IRES elements have distinct secondary, or even tertiary, structures that facilitate their function.

The plasmid bacterial backbone contains a prokaryotic origin of replication and the selection marker.

Plasmids are synthesized in their bacterial hosts, usually *E. coli* bacteria, as supercoiled circular DNA; however, a relaxed form caused by a nick on one strand can often be detected in purified plasmid preparations. In typical bacterial hosts, such as *E. coli*, dimers and even multimers are formed, which are caused by homologous recombination. This might be a concern for gene therapy applications, for which a homogeneous composition of the gene therapy drug is required. Hence, modifications in the single bacterial chromosome have been engineered in laboratory-used bacterial plasmid producers. To avoid multimer formation during plasmid preparation, the plasmids are produced in a bacterial strain that is deficient in the recombinase protein RecA. A deficiency in RecA can reduce the frequency of multimerization, and in some cases, it may completely prevent the formation of plasmid multimers. A supplementary strategy consists of inserting the parABCDE' locus from plasmid RK2 in the plasmid, thereby reducing the number of dimers formed. The parA gene encodes a resolvase that catalyzes recombination at the multimer resolution site in the parABCDE' locus. In addition, the parABCDE' locus helps ensure that plasmids are evenly distributed to daughter cells during cell division, which is essential for maintaining plasmid stability in bacterial populations.

The principle of plasmid exclusion, also known as incompatibility, is a phenomenon observed in bacteria where two plasmids that belong to the same incompatibility group cannot stably coexist in the same cell. This is because they use identical replication and partitioning mechanisms, leading to competition among the plasmids. As a result, one single plasmid, representing a monoclonal, homogeneous molecular entity, is found within bacterial expansion cultures.

High copy numbers of plasmids in each *E. coli* bacterial host cell are required to obtain reasonable amounts of plasmids that are devoid of contaminating bacterial chromosomal DNA and endotoxins. Most cloning plasmid vectors possess the ColE1 origin of replication, which has a well-understood mechanism of replication that involves the interaction between a plasmid-encoded sense-antisense RNA pair, RNA-I and RNA-II.

The RNA-II hybridizes to a strand of the ColE1 gene, thus creating a RNA–DNA heteroduplex which is cleaved by an enzyme called RNase H. This creates a 3'OH end, being used as a primer by the bacterial DNA polymerase, leading to the replication of the plasmid. Lagging strand synthesis is later initiated by a primase encoded by the host cell. The number of plasmids present within a single bacterial cell is regulated by the antisense RNA-I, which binds to the 5' end of RNA-II. This alters the folding of RNA-II, so that the DNA–RNA hybrid is not stabilized, and cleavage does not occur. This ensures that, at high copy numbers, replication is slowed down due to increased RNA-I concentration. The level of antisense transcript is proportional to the number of plasmids, creating a negative feedback loop that keeps plasmid copy number constant under specific conditions. In order to increase the number of plasmids in the bacterial host, a high-copy-number, modified origin of replication has been engineered, such as pUC21, whose ColE1 *ori* is protected from the RNA-II effect by mutating its RNA-II complementary sequence.

The delivery of plasmids to eukaryotic cells is described in Chapters 6 and 7. It has been shown that gene transfer efficacy is inversely proportional to the size of the plasmid: a much higher transfection efficacy is observed with smaller plasmids than with larger ones. This, along with regulatory considerations aiming at avoiding the use of antibiotic resistance genes, has prompted the development of minicircles and miniplasmids.

## 5.2 Minicircles and Miniplasmids: Clinical Applications

Plasmids currently used in preclinical and clinical trials contain a prokaryotic origin of replication and an antibiotic resistance gene; both, however, are undesirable for various reasons. One reason is that delivering the plasmid to patients for clinical use could lead to the dissemination of prokaryotic replicative recombinant DNA within them; endogenous enterobacteria, in which such plasmids could replicate, may acquire recombinant DNA, resulting in the uncontrolled dissemination of therapeutic and antibiotic resistance genes. These recombinant bacteria might then have a selective advantage, particularly if the corresponding antibiotic is administered. Also, antibiotic contamination during plasmid preparation is a concern when plasmids are delivered *in vivo* to patients, as it may lead to potential antibiotic allergic reactions.

Moreover, prokaryotic sequences can have other undesirable effects. For instance, antibodies have been produced against a prokaryotic endotoxin following the injection of a Bacillus thuringiensis plasmid carrying an endotoxin gene, expressed from cryptic upstream eukaryotic expression signals. In addition, short immunostimulatory DNA sequences containing CpG dinucleotides are present in the prokaryotic backbone of plasmids. These CpG sequences function as adjuvants for the immunogenic properties of plasmids encoding antigens in genetic immunization protocols. However, this effect is clearly undesirable for other applications where immune stimulation is not required. Finally, it has been shown that the antibiotic resistance selection marker can be detected in recombinant viral vectors which had been prepared by transfecting plasmids bearing such an antibiotic resistance gene (Chapters 3 to 5).

For the above-mentioned reasons, new-generation non-viral DNA vectors have been developed to meet the requirements of regulatory agencies that recommend avoiding the use of antibiotics during the manufacturing process, whenever possible, and thus the removal of antibiotic resistance selection markers from the plasmid backbone. In addition, deleting the antibiotic resistance selection markers allows decreasing the vector size, thereby improving transfection efficacy.

Several approaches for safer plasmids have been implemented to achieve that aim. The first strategy uses an *in cellulo* recombination step in order to separate the bacterial backbone from the transcription cassette; this separation occurs within the bacterial host. This recombination must be triggered at the end of the expansion culture, immediately before the lysis of the bacterial host cells and subsequent purification. This process releases two circular DNA molecules: the expression cassette, circularized into a "minicircle", and the bacterial backbone alone, circularized into a "miniplasmid" (Figure 5.2).

In the example shown in Figure 5.2, a supercoiled DNA minicircle is produced by *in vivo* site-specific recombination. The minicircle contains exclusively the desired, excisable fragment. Site-specific recombination is driven by bacteriophage lambda integrase in a parental plasmid containing the 530bp attP site of bacteriophage lamda (also called phage lambda). and the 31 bp *E. coli* minimal attB sequence in the same orientation. The minicircle is the product of *in cellulo* excision of the desired cassette by site-specific intramolecular recombination between the attP and attB sequences. This excision/recombination is driven by *E. coli* bacteriophage integrase. The expression of the integrase is triggered by a temperature jump from 37°C to 42°C. This initial system has been refined by several teams. A decatenation step between the minicircle and the miniplasmid is obtained by the action of the *E. coli* DNA topoisomerase IV.

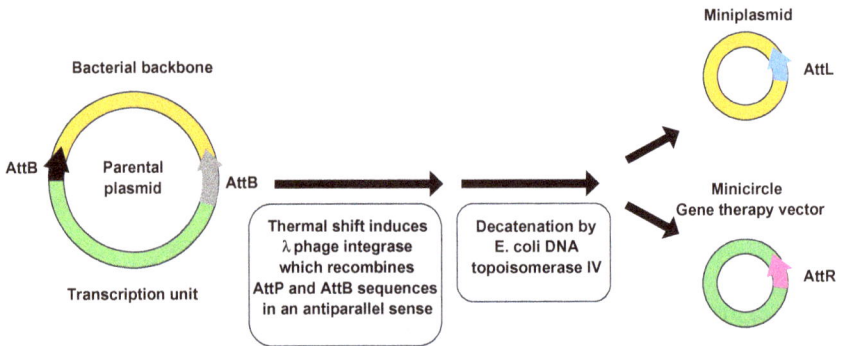

**Figure 5.2.**   The bacterial host is equipped with a λ phage integrase which is under a thermosensitive repressor. Upon a thermal jump from 37°C to 42°C, the integrase is expressed. Recombination leads to the production of the minicircle and miniplasmid, which are decatenated by the *E. coli* DNA topoisomerase IV. Other induction tools can be used for activating the integrase at the end of the expansion culture, such as the lactose operon system (the lac operator and lac repressor are key components of the lac operon, a gene regulatory system in *E. coli* and other bacteria that controls the metabolism of lactose).

Several other systems, apart from those using *in cellulo* recombination, have been introduced. Their use is increasing. They all aim at providing a selection pressure, which is independent of the use of any antibiotic, to maintain the plasmid at a high copy number in the bacterial host *E. coli*. They are reviewed by Scherman and Marie (2024). They include the pCOR, nanoplasmids, GenCircle, and pORT systems.

As the first described example of all these plasmid families, the pCOR backbone possesses several features that increase safety in terms of dissemination and selection, as follows: (1) the plasmid's selectable marker is not an antibiotic resistance gene but a gene encoding a bacterial suppressor tRNA; and (2) the origin of replication requires a plasmid-specific initiator protein, the π protein, encoded by the *pir* gene, thus limiting its host range to bacterial strains that produce this trans-acting protein. Optimized *E. coli* hosts supporting pCOR replication and selection led to the production of high yields (up to 100 mg/L) of supercoiled pCOR monomers through fed-batch fermentation. The NV1FGF pCOR plasmid has been used in a phase III multicenter clinical trial to treat intermittent claudication and critical limb ischemia. The NV1FGF plasmid, a pCOR plasmid, carries the angiogenic fibroblast growth factor (FGF) cDNA sequence, which was injected into the skeletal muscles.

The example of the plasmid family pFAR (plasmid free of antibiotic resistance gene), displayed in Figure 5.3, uses the principle of auxotrophy. A stop codon is introduced in the *E. coli* chromosomal gene involved in the synthesis of the DNA component thymidine. In consequence, the bacteria cannot grow in a culture medium devoid of this particular nucleic base because they cannot synthesize it. The plasmid is then engineered in order to carry a tRNA which hybridizes with the stop codon sequence, thereby overcoming the stop mutation and enabling the *in cellulo* synthesis of the missing nucleic base by functional thymidylate synthase enzyme. This strategy confers selection pressure because the bacterial host must maintain the plasmid carrying the tRNA in order to grow. In the plasmids of the pFAR family, the stop codon renders the bacterial host auxotrophic for the base thymidine. This is illustrated in Figure 5.4.

✓ **small size: 1.1 kb**
✓ **reduced CpG content**
✓ **contains a multiple cloning site MCS**

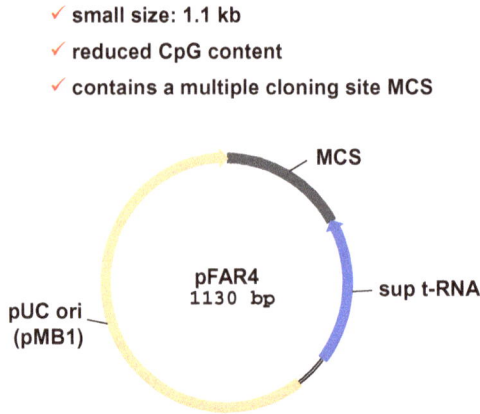

**Figure 5.3.**   The pFAR family: plasmids free of antibiotic resistance marker.

A first-in-man gene therapy clinical trial seeking to improve the hearing capacity of patients receiving a cochlear implant was launched in 2022 using a plasmid carrying the brain-derived neurotrophic factor (BDNF) gene and the neurotrophin 3 (NT3) gene. Cochlear implants consist of a set of miniaturized electrodes which stimulate spiral auditory neurons. Since each electrode corresponds to a given sound frequency, this allows the reconstitution by the auditory spiral nerve of part of the sound signal. This reconstitution, however, is imperfect in severe hearing disorders because of degenerated spiral sensory neurons that have lost their axons, which would normally be in contact with the cochlear hair cells. Hence, there is a spatial gap between the cochlear implant electrodes and hearing sensory neurons. The gene therapy approach aims at inducing the growth of spiral nerve neurons toward the cochlear implant through the local production of neurotrophins BDNF and NT3.

It was found in preclinical studies that the pFAR plasmid was taken up by the mesenchymal cells lining the cochlear fluid compartment when electrical pulses were delivered to a cochlear implant array reconfigured to produce a highly focused electric field. This "electrotransfer" process is described in Chapter 7. The electrotransfected cochlear mesenchymal cells

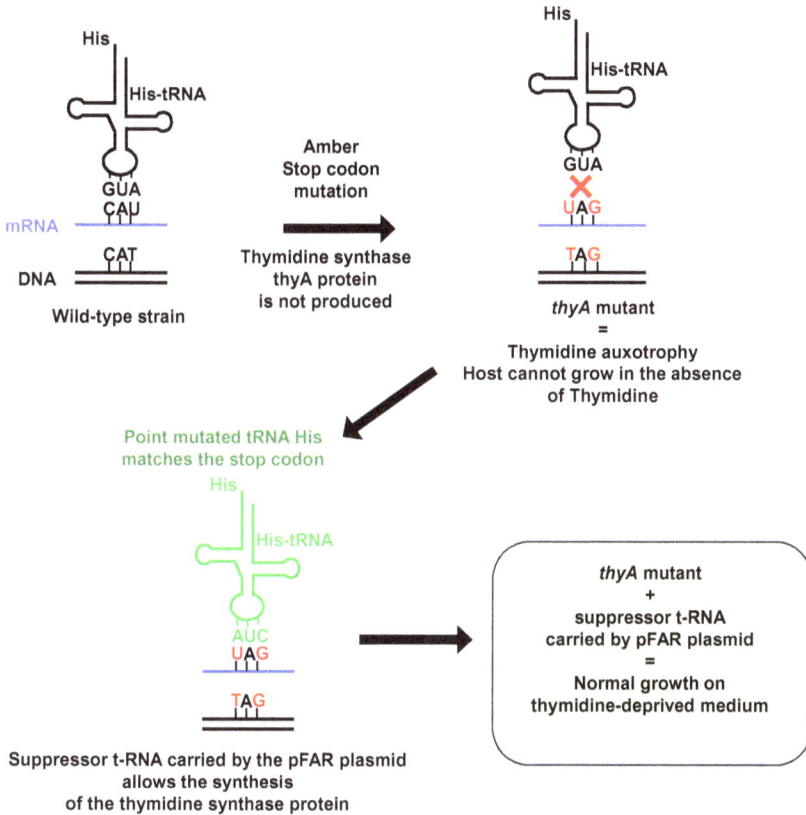

**Figure 5.4.** Principle of the biosafe pFAR plasmid. A stop codon is inserted within the coding sequence of the *E. coli thyA* thymidylate synthase gene. Consequently, the engineered bacterial host does not grow in a medium devoid of thymidine. Growth is allowed thanks to the pFAR plasmid encoding a tRNA matching the stop codon and allowing the proper addition of the amino acid histidine during *thyA* mRNA translation to protein. The bacterial host can then synthesize thymidine and grow in a thymidine-free culture medium. The tRNA, encoded by the pFAR plasmid, is called an amber mutation suppressor.

produce a localized concentration of neurotrophic factors, thus providing a directional stimulus for the regrowth of neuron axonal fibers. This leads to close contact between the spiral nerve dendrites and the cochlear implant array aiming at improving hearing performance (Figure 5.5). The phase I human clinical trial led to encouraging positive results.

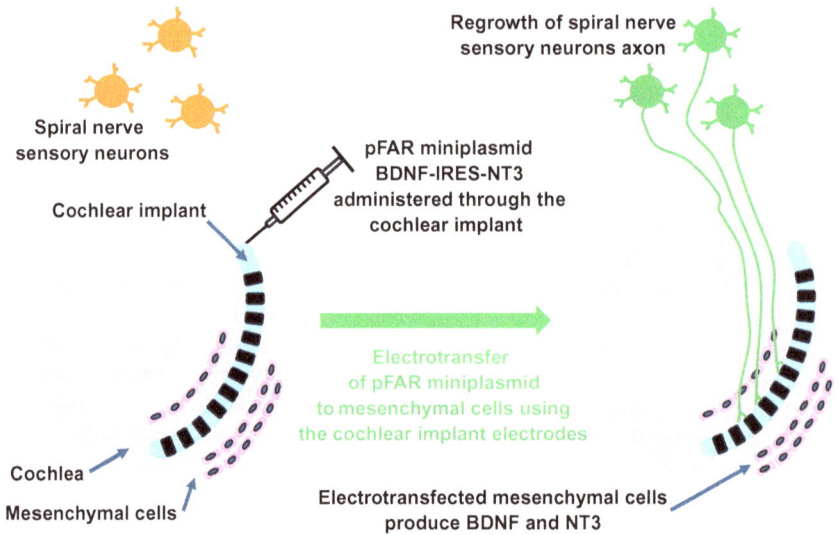

**Figure 5.5.** Schematic diagram depicting the axon regrowth of the auditory spiral nerve sensory neurons in response to BDNF and NT3 secreted locally by cochlear mesenchymal cells. The expression vector, pFAR4-CMVp-BDNF-IRES-NT3, carries BDNF and NT3 cDNA sequences under the cytomegalovirus promoter. The BDNF and NT3 cDNA sequences are separated by an IRES, which allows for the translation of the two proteins from a single mRNA (Section 5.1).

## 5.3  Linear DNA and Synthetic DNA Vectors

A more recent technology has been introduced as a potential replacement for circular plasmids. Cell-free long DNA synthesis can produce linear DNA using appropriate substrates, DNA polymerase, and other enzymes. The main advantage is that only necessary eukaryotic sequences, consisting of the expression cassette (promoter, gene, and poly(A)) are synthesized, thus preventing the presence of exogenous prokaryotic bacterial DNA sequences. It is not clear at the present time if this *in vitro* synthetic production system leads to equivalent or even superior transgene expression because DNA supercoiling, which is observed in plasmids, is considered to be necessary to promote intracellular DNA stability and transcription. Different systems have been introduced, such as the Doggybone or MIDGE systems.

Doggybone DNA (dbDNA) is a minimal, linear, double-stranded, and covalently closed DNA construct. For Doggybone production, a circular plasmid DNA template is chemically denatured. Rolling circle amplification using Φ29 DNA polymerase and primers produces long, linear concatemers. Then, recombinant pro-telomerase binds the linear DNA at specific sites, creating dbDNA. Minimal immunologically defined gene expression (MIDGE) vectors consist of an expression cassette flanked by two short hairpin oligonucleotide sequences. They are manufactured from plasmids which are specifically designed for the excision of the entire expression cassette and subsequent ligation of short hairpin oligodeoxy-nucleotides by an enzymatic process.

## 5.4 Transposons for Transgene Integration

Plasmids transfected into eukaryotic cells remain episomal in the nucleus, which means that the transgene is not integrated into the host cells' chromosomes. When cells divide, such as tumor cells, hematopoietic stem cells, or during tissue regeneration, these episomal plasmids are lost upon cell mitosis and daughter cell segregation. It is, therefore, important for these dividing cell types to achieve stable transfection through the integration of the transgene into the genome of the host. This is made possible by the use of oncoretroviruses or lentiviruses, as described in Chapter 4. This is also possible in a non-viral gene therapy context by using the transposon machinery, which allows stable integration of plasmid-carried transgenes into the host cells' chromosomes. This has been used, for instance, for the non-viral generation of CAR-T cells in adoptive immunotherapy, thus avoiding the use of lentiviral vectors (Chapter 8).

Transposons are mobile genetic elements evolved to execute highly efficient integration of their genes into the genomes of their host cells. These natural DNA transfer vehicles have been adapted and optimized to stably introduce foreign DNA sequences into the genomes of target cells in a regulated and highly efficient manner. Transposon systems are recognized tools for genetic engineering, basic research applications such as mutagenesis screens to discover gene functions, and gene therapy approaches in both preclinical and clinical settings.

The most basic mechanism of natural transposon movement is "cut-and-paste" transposition, during which a transposase enzyme mediates the excision of the element from its donor location and its reintegration into a new chromosomal locus. This allows the transposons to "travel over the genome". During transposition, the transposase interacts with its binding sites on the DNA inverted terminal repeats (ITRs), which define the boundaries of the transposon. This promotes the assembly of a synaptic complex, also called paired-end complex (PEC). The transposase dimers then catalyze the excision of the element from its donor site and integrate the excised transposon into a new location within the chromosomal DNA.

The three amino acids aspartate–aspartate–glutamate (DDE), coordinated with Mg++ ions, play an essential role in the excision/integration catalytic mechanism. The key biochemical process of all transposon excision reactions executed by DDE recombinases involves the exposure by a single-stranded nick of 3'OH groups at the transposon ends, which is subsequently used during the strand transfer reaction for integration. During cut-and-paste transposition, nicking of the element is followed by the cleavage of the complementary DNA strand, resulting in a double-strand break (DSB) that liberates the transposon from the donor DNA.

The three most frequently used transposon systems for gene therapy and laboratory applications are the Sleeping Beauty (SB; Figure 5.6), the piggyBac, and the Tol2 transposon systems. The mechanism of transposition is different for each of these systems. For instance, the SB system shows a nearly random integration profile in mammalian genomes. The excision site is primarily repaired by non-homologous end joining, thereby leaving behind a characteristic CAG footprint originating from the terminal sequences of the SB transposon, which remain at the excision site after cleavage by the transposase. On the contrary, The PiggyBac transposon possess the unique capacity to excise DNA without leaving behind a footprint in the genome. This feature makes PiggyBac a popular choice for applications where a "clean" removal of the inserted DNA is necessary.

The SB transposon system uses inverted repeats/direct repeats (IR/DRs) as key elements for its function. These IR/DRs are sequences

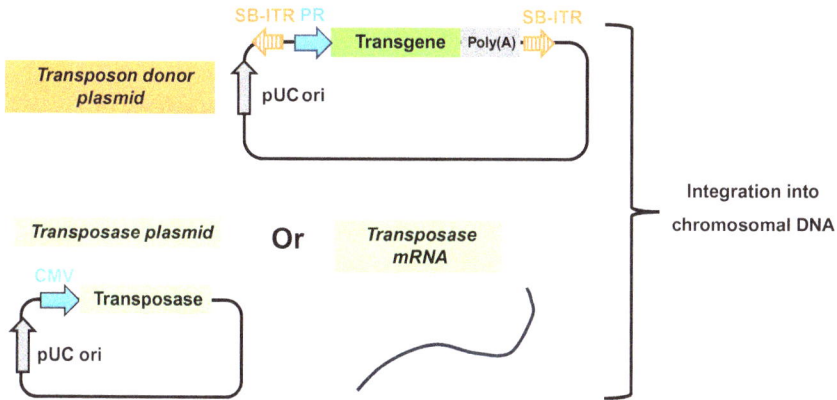

**Figure 5.6.** Sleeping Beauty (SB) transposase-mediated transposition through a cut-and-paste mechanism for non-viral gene therapy. A GOI (bright green upper bar) under either a ubiquitous or tissue-specific promoter (PR) is borne by a transposon donor plasmid. The transposase can be delivered via a transposase gene carried by a plasmid controlled by a strong promoter such as CMV. Alternatively, the transposase can be delivered as an mRNA molecule which shows several advantages: (1) mRNA does not have to be delivered to the nucleus but only needs to reach the cytosol, which is much easier to obtain; (2) most importantly, this allows the transposase to be transient, which is crucial, because the transposase has nuclease capacity and could be detrimental to the host genome.

that flank the transposon and are recognized by the SB transposase enzyme. The IRs are sequences of DNA that are inverted and repeated on either side of the transposon. The DRs are sequences that are repeated in the same direction. The transposase enzyme binds to these IR/DRs, excises the transposon from its original location, and integrates it into a new site in the genome, typically at a TA dinucleotide site (Figure 5.7). A transposase dimer binds to both ITRs in the transposon donor plasmid and forms a tetramer, which leads to the integration of the GOI into the host genome. The transposase possesses a nuclear localization sequence (NLS), two DNA-binding domains, and a C-terminal catalytic domain with nuclease activity. In contrast to retroviruses, the SB transposase does not target actively transcribed chromosomal sites, which renders it safer in terms of insertional oncogenesis risk.

The piggyBac transposon originates in the insect genome and is active in a large variety of cells, such as yeast, plant, non-human mammal, and

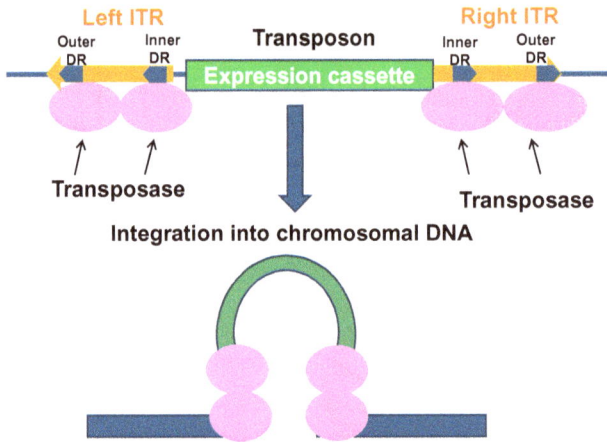

**Figure 5.7.** Mechanism of SB transposon genomic insertion. The transposase binds to the terminal inverted repeats, induces double-stranded breaks (indicated by yellow lightning bolts), and excises the mobile element from the donor DNA, leaving behind a footprint. The transposon–transposase complex identifies a suitable target site (a TA nucleotide) and performs integration.

human cells. In contrast to SB's preference to integrate into TA dinucleotides, the piggyBac transposon preferentially integrates into TTAA sequences, which are duplicated during insertion, thereby flanking the inserted transposon. Also, in contrast to the SB transposon, piggyBac displays a preference for integration near transcriptional start sites, similar to gamma oncoretroviruses.

As mentioned above, a distinctive and highly attractive feature of the piggyBac transposase is that, in contrast to most transposases, its excision leaves no footprint behind at a transposase-mediated transposon excision site, which is interesting for laboratory applications. This does not represent a decisive advantage for most gene therapy applications, however, since transposons are used for the stable integration of therapeutic transgenes, with limited or no excision events. However, this property is advantageous in certain cases when only a transient expression of a transgene is required, such as when introducing reprogramming factors into somatic cells to generate induced pluripotent stem cells (iPSCs). In such cases, obtaining an excision-only piggyBac transposase mutant allows deleting the transiently expressed transgene without any footprint, thus avoiding the risk of frame-shift mutations.

The Tol2 transposons are less frequently used compared to SB and piggyBac. The Tol2 target site selection is less defined, with a weak consensus palindromic-like TNA (C/G)TTATAA(G/C)TNA octanucleotide sequence. The Tol2 transposon generates an 8 bp target site duplication at the integration sites. Tol2 has been used in the generation of transgenic animals (mouse, chicken, frog, and zebrafish models) and to generate insertional mutagenesis.

## 5.5 mRNA as Gene Expression Vector for Therapy and Vaccines

mRNA vectors represent the most recently introduced gene therapy vectors. Their development has been delayed due to several difficulties concerning their production, maintenance, and strong immunoinflammatory properties, which are now resolved. The structure of an mRNA is composed of a 5' cap, a 5' untranslated region (5' UTR), an open reading frame encoding the mature sequence of the protein to be translated, and a 3' untranslated region (3' UTR) terminated by a poly(A) tail (Figure 5.8).

The cap structure at the 5' end of mRNA is critical for the efficient translation, stabilization, and transport of mRNAs in eukaryotes. The capping of mRNA is highly regulated and essential for creating stable, mature messenger RNA capable of undergoing translation during protein synthesis, as it promotes mRNA entry into the ribosomal machinery. In eukaryotes, the cap is recognized by the eukaryotic initiation factor 4E (eIF4E). After eIF4E binding, eIF4E then recruits the scaffold protein eIF4G, which in turn brings the RNA helicase eIF4A to the mRNA. The helicase eIF4A unwinds secondary structures in the 5' UTR of the mRNA, facilitating the recruitment of the ribosomal 40S subunit pre-initiation

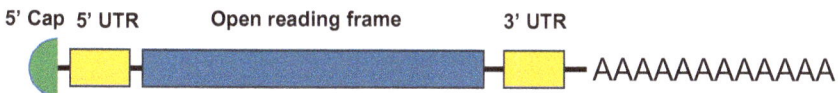

5' Cap 5' UTR    Open reading frame    3' UTR

AAAAAAAAAAAA

**Figure 5.8.** mRNA structure.

complex. This complex, which includes the small ribosomal subunit, scans the mRNA until it finds the start codon, initiating translation.

The 5' cap in eukaryotes consists of a guanine nucleotide connected to mRNA via an unusual 5'–5' triphosphate linkage. This guanosine is methylated on the seventh position directly after capping *in vivo* by the enzyme guanine-N7-)-methyltransferase using S-adenosylmethionine as substrate, a universal methyl group donor. This cap is referred to as a 7-methylguanylate cap, abbreviated to m7G. This represents the simplest Cap structure, which is called CAP-0, and occurs on mRNA molecules transcribed by RNA polymerase II. In multicellular eukaryotes and some viruses, further modifications exist, including the methylation of the 2' hydroxy-groups of the first two ribose sugars at the 5' end of the mRNA, leading to the variants Cap 1 and Cap 2 (Figure 5.9).

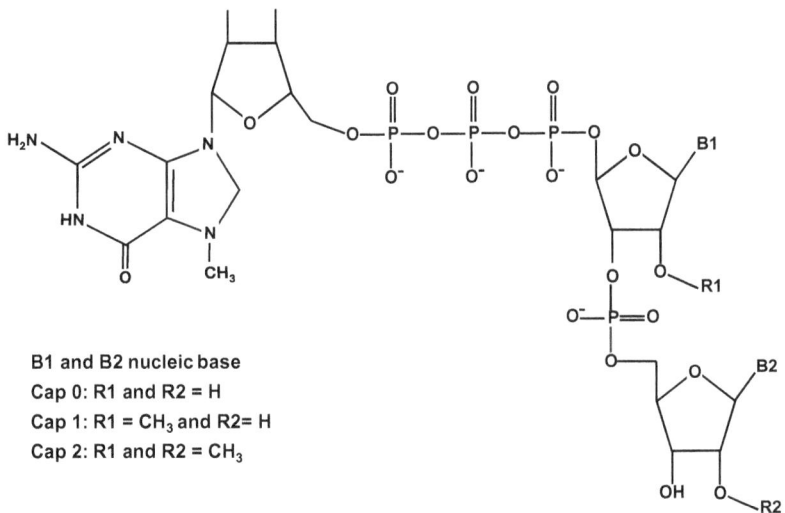

**Figure 5.9.**   Chemical structure of Cap 0, Cap1, and Cap 2. The capping process is initiated before the completion of transcription, while the nascent pre-mRNA is being synthesized. One of the terminal phosphate groups is removed by RNA triphosphatase, leaving a bisphosphate group. Then, GTP is added to the terminal bisphosphate by mRNA guanylyltransferase, losing a pyrophosphate from the GTP substrate in the process. This results in the 5'–5' triphosphate linkage. The seventh nitrogen of guanine is then methylated by the mRNA (guanine-N7-)-methyltransferase. In addition, there are further methylations of the first bases of the mRNA at position 2' of the ribose, leading to Cap1 (only the first base being methylated) or Cap2 (the first two bases being methylated).

In the perspective of mRNA therapy and vaccines, multiple chemical modifications have been introduced into the Cap in order to increase mRNA stability and enhance ribosomal engagement, leading to enhanced transcription rate and efficacy.

The 5' UTR in mRNA is the region directly upstream from the initiation codon. This region is important for the regulation of the translation of a transcript through differing mechanisms in viruses, prokaryotes, and eukaryotes. While it is called untranslated, the 5' UTR, or part of it, is sometimes translated into a protein product. This product can then regulate the translation of the main mRNA coding sequence. In many organisms, however, the 5' UTR is completely untranslated; instead, it forms a complex secondary mRNA structure to regulate translation.

The 5' UTR begins at the transcription start site and ends one nucleotide before the initiation sequence (usually AUG) of the coding region. In prokaryotes, the length of the 5' UTR typically ranges from 3 to 10 nucleotides, whereas in eukaryotes it varies widely, extending from about 100 to several thousand nucleotides. The prokaryotic 5' UTR contains a ribosome-binding site (RBS), also known as the Shine–Dalgarno sequence (AGGAGGU), which is usually 3–10 base pairs upstream of the initiation codon. In contrast, the eukaryotic 5' UTR contains the Kozak consensus sequence (ACCAUGG), which contains the initiation codon. These are general characteristics, and the exact sequence of the 5' UTR can vary greatly depending on the specific gene and organism.

The open reading frame between the 5' UTR and 3' UTR is the coding sequence (CDS) containing start and stop codons.

The 3' UTR of mRNA follows the translation termination codon. It plays significant roles in the regulation of gene expression. The 3' UTR contains binding sites for regulatory proteins and microRNAs (miRNAs). These elements can influence mRNA stability, localization, and translation efficiency. The 3' UTR contains sequences rich in adenine (A) and uridine (U) AU-rich elements (AREs), which are involved in the regulation of mRNA decay. The sequence AAUAAA within the 3' UTR directs the addition of a poly(A) tail, which is important for mRNA stability and translation. Finally, the 3' UTR physical characteristics, such as length and secondary structures, also contribute to its regulatory functions.

The average length of the 3' UTR in humans is approximately 800 nucleotides; however, it can vary significantly.

The polyadenylate (poly(A)) tail is a crucial component of messenger RNA (mRNA) in eukaryotes. It stabilizes the mRNA molecule and prevents its degradation. The poly(A) tail can function synergistically with the (m7G) cap to stimulate translation, independently of its length. It also allows the mature mRNA molecule to be exported from the nucleus and translated into a protein by ribosomes in the cytoplasm. Globally, the poly(A) tail has the ability to recruit RNA-binding proteins and then interact with diverse factors to send various signals to regulate mRNA metabolism. The length of the poly(A) tail can influence the efficiency of translation.

In summary, the basic structure of *in vitro*-transcribed mRNA vectors includes a 5' cap, a 5' UTR, a coding sequence containing start and stop codons, a 3' UTR, and a poly(A) tail. These mRNA features are all necessary to create a loop structure via the poly(A)-binding protein (PABP), enabling efficient translation. The loop structure and mRNA translation process is schematized in Figure 5.10. A modified nucleoside, such as pseudouridine, is often used to suppress immunogenicity in the host cells (Section 5.6).

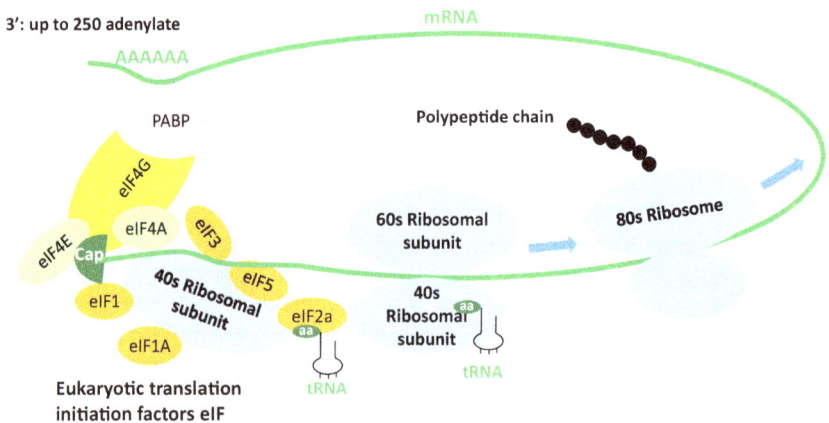

**Figure 5.10.**   mRNA loop and translation process.

## 5.6　Control of Undesired Innate Immune System Activation by Exogenous mRNA

mRNA can induce an innate immune response through its interaction with pattern recognition receptors (PRRs), including Toll-like receptors (TLRs). This is because the immune system recognizes foreign mRNA as a potential threat, similar to viral RNA. Specifically, structured elements within the mRNA UTRs may form secondary structures that induce TLR-3 signaling. Moreover, GU-enriched RNA sequences, sensed by TLR7/8, can drive the production of proinflammatory cytokines, including TNF-$\alpha$, IL-6, and IFN$\gamma$.

This immune response can be a double-edged sword. While it could be beneficial for activating the immune response to genetic vaccines, it is, in fact, much more detrimental as it indirectly blocks mRNA translation. This can lead to reduced efficacy of mRNA vaccines and therapies and may potentially cause immune-related side effects. This detrimental effect has been controlled by the use of pseudouridine (Figure 5.11), which represents the most abundant RNA modification in mammals. When incorporated into mRNA, pseudouridine reduces the inflammatory

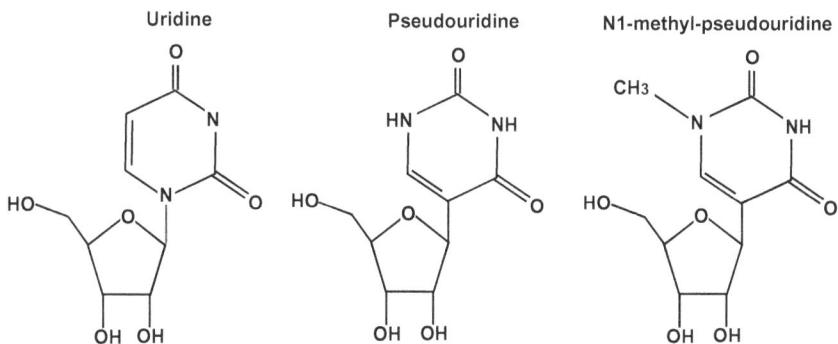

**Figure 5.11.** Chemical formula of uridine, pseudouridine, and N1-methyl-pseudouridine.

and innate immunity response against mRNA. This is achieved by making the mRNA appear more "self", or human-like, so that the body generates an immune response to the encoded antigen rather than simply destroying the mRNA.

Pseudouridine replacement has been crucial in the development of mRNA vaccines, such as those against the virus SARS-CoV-2 responsible for COVID-19. These vaccines are based on mRNA encoding the spike protein of the virus. In the two mRNA vaccines against SARS-CoV-2, Comirnaty and Spikevax, uridine is replaced by N1-methyl-pseudouridine. This modification is believed to contribute to the high efficacy of these vaccines by reducing the innate immune response against mRNA itself. In contrast, mRNA vaccines developed by other teams and using unmodified mRNA showed lower efficacy.

In summary, pseudouridine or pseudouridine derivatives introduced in mRNA in replacement of uridine can help balance the innate immune response, thereby improving the efficacy and safety of mRNA-based therapies and vaccines. However, more research is needed to fully understand the role of pseudouridine and other RNA modifications in mRNA immunogenicity and potency.

## 5.7  Clinical Applications of mRNA Vectors

The mRNA vaccines against SARS-CoV-2, Comirnaty and Spikevax, have been administered to hundreds of millions of patients. This has paved the way for the active development of other vaccine candidates. Vaccines against influenza viruses, respiratory syncytial virus (RSV), cytomegalovirus (CMV), and Epstein–Barr virus (EBV), as well as combination vaccines, are under development. Cancer vaccines also show promising perspectives.

In addition, continuous updates of the SARS-CoV-2 vaccines to better protect against mutated variants of the virus are being produced, and several strategies have been found to improve the efficiency of

COVID-19 mRNA vaccines, such as mutating two proline codons to stabilize the S protein translation product or using modified mRNA encoding prefusion S protein.

A key advantage of mRNA vaccines is that an efficient formulation is identical for all mRNA vaccines, independent of the mRNA sequence. This is in contrast to inactivated virus vaccines and classical protein subunit vaccines, for which a specific formulation must be tailored for each case. As soon as the genetic sequence of a new virus is identified, available software programs help to identify optimal mRNA sequences for the vaccine candidate, and ready-to-use formulations can be employed. This represents a crucial advantage in terms of speed and cost.

For gene therapy, mRNA drugs are also progressing. Cellular mRNA lifetime is much shorter than DNA. This represents a major hurdle for gene therapy, but can be considered valuable in some applications. Some mRNAs are under clinical investigation, such as mRNA-3705, developed for the treatment of methylmalonic acidemia (MMA), a rare and life-threatening inherited metabolic disorder. MMA is most commonly caused by a deficiency in the mitochondrial enzyme methylmalonic-CoA mutase (MUT), leading to the toxic buildup of acids in the body and resulting in severe health issues. The mRNA of the deficient enzyme is inserted into a lipid nucleoparticle and is IV administered for liver delivery (see Chapter 6 for more details on LNP lipid nanoparticle technology). Other applications for cardiac diseases are also being developed.

An interesting actively developed mRNA drug is the LNP mRNA formulation to express darbepoetin for the treatment of anemia due to chronic kidney disease (CKD) and to non-myeloid malignancies where anemia is due to the effect of concomitant myelosuppressive chemotherapy. While recombinant protein erythropoietin (EPO) is available to patients, the price of the treatment could be reduced more than 10-fold if this could be replaced by an mRNA, whose production costs are considered to be much lower than those of recombinant proteins.

## 5.8  Production of mRNA Vectors

For COVID19 vaccines, mRNA is selected and produced through the following steps:

(1) Design the mRNA sequence by identifying the target (virus's spike protein for SARS-CoV-2) for generating a protective immune response. This sequence is then optimized for stability and efficiency.

(2) Synthesis of the corresponding double-strand DNA inserted into a plasmid, which serves as a template for mRNA production (synthetic DNA might also be used).

(3) *In vitro* transcription to mRNA using the T7 RNA polymerase. This enzyme is highly efficient and specific for *in vitro* transcription (IVT) reactions. The reaction is performed at a temperature between 37°C and 50°C in a buffered medium in the presence of 0.25 mM ethylenediaminetetraacetic acid (EDTA; a cation complexation agent). EDTA plays a crucial role in mRNA production by acting as a chelating agent. EDTA binds to divalent metal ions, such as magnesium ($Mg^{2+}$) and calcium ($Ca^{2+}$). This helps prevent the degradation of DNA and RNA by inactivating nucleases that require these metal ions for catalytic reaction. Also, EDTA helps maintain the stability of the reaction environment, which is essential for efficient mRNA synthesis. In addition, the reaction mixture contains a detergent (Tween-20), an RNase inhibitor, and inorganic pyrophosphatase. Optimally, it is possible to generate milligram quantities of mRNA from microgram amounts of plasmid DNA. This translates to billions of mRNA molecules, given that 1 mg of mRNA consists of approximately $10^{12}$ molecules.

(4) Capping can be performed either co-transcriptionally using a Cap analog reactant, or post-transcriptionally using the Vaccinia capping enzyme, which adds a guanosine cap to the 5' end of the mRNA, and 2'-O-Methyltransferase, which methylates the first nucleotide adjacent to the cap to form a cap-1 structure.

(5) *Purification*: The resulting mRNA is purified to remove any contaminants or unwanted by-products.

(6) *Encapsulation in lipid nanoparticles*: mRNA is fragile and needs protection to ensure effective delivery into human cells. It is

encapsulated in lipid nanoparticles, which help protect the mRNA and facilitate its entry into cells.

(7) *Quality control and testing*: The final product undergoes rigorous quality control and testing to ensure its safety, efficacy, and purity.

This process allows for rapid and scalable production of mRNA vaccines, which was crucial in responding to the COVID-19 pandemic.

## Acknowledgment

We wish to thank Dr. Corinne Marie for her contribution to the section on pFAR vectors.

## Bibliography

Borja GM, Meza Mora E, Barrón B, Gosset G, Ramírez OT, Lara AR. Engineering Escherichia coli to increase plasmid DNA production in high cell-density cultivations in batch mode. *Microb Cell Fact*. 2012 Sep;11:132. doi: 10.1186/1475-2859-11-132.

Boussif O, Lezoualc'h F, Zanta MA, Mergny MD, Scherman D, Demeneix B, Behr JP. A versatile vector for gene and oligonucleotide transfer into cells in culture and in vivo: polyethylenimine. *Proc Natl Acad Sci U S A*. 1995 Aug;92(16):7297–301. doi: 10.1073/pnas.92.16.7297.

Darquet AM, Rangara R, Kreiss P, Schwartz B, Naimi S, Delaère P, Crouzet J, Scherman D. Minicircle: an improved DNA molecule for in vitro and in vivo gene transfer. *Gene Ther*. 1999 Feb;6(2):209–18. doi: 10.1038/sj.gt.3300816.

Hayes F. The function and organization of plasmids. In: Casali N, Presto A, editors. *E. Coli Plasmid Vectors: Methods and Applications. Methods in Molecular Biology*. Vol. 235. Humana Press; 2003. p. 1–5.

Karikó K, Muramatsu H, Welsh FA, Ludwig J, Kato H, Akira S, Weissman D. Incorporation of pseudouridine into mRNA yields superior nonimmunogenic vector with increased translational capacity and biological stability. *Mol Ther*. 2008 Nov;16(11):1833–40. doi: 10.1038/mt.2008.200.

Marie C, Scherman D. Antibiotic-free gene vectors: a 25-year journey to clinical trials. *Genes*. 2024 Feb;15(3):261. doi: 10.3390/genes15030261.

Pardi N, Weissman D. Nucleoside modified mRNA vaccines for infectious diseases. *Methods Mol Biol*. 2017;1499:109–121. doi: 10.1007/978-1-4939-6481-9_6.

Parhiz H, Atochina-Vasserman EN, Weissman D. mRNA-based therapeutics: looking beyond COVID-19 vaccines. *Lancet.* 2024 Mar;403(10432):1192–1204. doi: 10.1016/S0140-6736(23)02444-3.

Pastor M, Quiviger M, Pailloux J, Scherman D, Marie C. Reduced heterochromatin formation on the pFAR4 miniplasmid allows sustained transgene expression in the mouse liver. *Mol Ther Nucleic Acids.* 2020 Sep;21:28–36. doi: 10.1016/j.omtn.2020.05.014.

Qin S, Tang X, Chen Y, *et al.* mRNA-based therapeutics: powerful and versatile tools to combat diseases. *Signal Transduct Target Ther.* 2022 May;7(1):166. doi: 10.1038/s41392-022-01007-w.

Sandoval-Villegas N, Nurieva W, Amberger M, Ivics Z. Contemporary transposon tools: a review and guide through mechanisms and applications of sleeping beauty, piggyBac and Tol2 for genome engineering. *Int J Mol Sci.* 2021 May;22(10):5084. doi: 10.3390/ijms22105084.

Schnödt M, Schmeer M, Kracher B, Krüsemann C, Espinosa LE, Grünert A, Fuchsluger T, Rischmüller A. DNA minicircle technology improves purity of adeno-associated viral vector preparations. *Mol Ther Nucleic Acids.* 2016;5(8):e355. doi: 10.1038/mtna.2016.60.

Thomas CM, Summers D. Bacterial plasmids. *Encyclopedia of Life Sciences.* 2008. doi: 10.1002/9780470015902.a0000468.pub2.

Vandermeulen G, Marie C, Scherman D, Préat V. New generation of plasmid backbones devoid of antibiotic resistance marker for gene therapy trials. *Mol Ther.* 2011 Nov;19(11):1942–9. doi: 10.1038/mt.2011.182.

Vavassori V, Ferrari S, Beretta S, Asperti C, Albano L, Annoni A, Gaddoni C, Varesi A. Lipid nanoparticles allow efficient and harmless ex vivo gene editing of human hematopoietic cells. *Blood.* 2023 Aug;142(9):812–826. doi: 10.1182/blood.2022019333.

Wang YS, Kumari M, Chen GH, Hong MH, Yuan JP, Tsai JL, Wu HC. mRNA-based vaccines and therapeutics: an in-depth survey of current and upcoming clinical applications. *J Biomed Sci.* 2023 Oct;30(1):84. doi: 10.1186/s12929-023-00977-5.

Weissman D. mRNA transcript therapy. *Expert Rev Vaccines.* 2015 Feb;14(2):265–81. doi: 10.1586/14760584.2015.973859.

Weissman D, Karikó K. mRNA: fulfilling the promise of gene therapy. *Mol Ther.* 2015 Sep;23(9):1416–7. doi: 10.1038/mt.2015.138.

# Chapter 6

# Chemical Delivery of Non-Viral Vectors

Quite significant barriers, as listed in the following, must be overcome in order to deliver to the cells mRNA, DNA, most antisense oligodeoxinucleotides (ASOs), and short silencing RNA (siRNA):

(1) First, these nucleic acids bear one phosphate negative charge per nucleotide and are thus polyanionic. Similarly, the cell plasma membrane bears a high density of negative charges which are mainly attributed not only to the phospholipid negative phosphate but also to the sialic acids and other carboxylate-bearing moieties present on glycolipids and glycoproteins at the external face of the external membrane of all cells. The negative charge of these cell membranes represents an electrostatic repulsion barrier against the passage and intracellular delivery of mRNA, DNA, ASOs, and siRNA.

(2) Second, intramolecular electrostatic repulsion between the negative phosphate groups leads to an extended shape of polynucleotides nucleic acids when suspended in aqueous media, making it unfavorable for crossing cell membranes.

(3) Third, the polyanionic nature of nucleotides contributes to their high degree of hydrophilicity, as opposed to the hydrophobic characteristic of the lipid bilayer membranes.

(4) Fourth, rapid degradation by extracellular endonucleases or exonucleases occurs.

(5) And fifth, short-sized antisense deoxynucleotides or silencing RNA (Chapters 10 and 11) undergo rapid renal elimination because their size is below the glomerular filtration limit.

The major hurdles caused by electrostatic repulsion between nucleotides and cell membrane, as well as by the cellular hydrophobicity barrier, have been tackled by associating the nucleotides with cationic vectors in order to form complexes called polyplexes, lipoplexes, or lipid nanoparticles (LNPs) (Sections 6.1–6.7). In addition, large DNA or mRNA molecules are compacted within these formulations because the positive charges brought about by the cationic delivery vectors counteract the electrostatic intramolecular repulsion forces. This drastically decreases their size in biological media.

Protection against endonucleases or exonucleases is also obtained through the formulation of lipoplexes, polyplexes, or LNPs. Finally, efficient delivery to the desired cells and renal filtration escape has shown great recent progress and therapeutic success; this will be described in Sections 6.7–6.9.

The process of delivering non-viral nucleic acids (mRNA, DNA, ASOs, and siRNA) is called cell transfection, in contrast to cell transduction mediated by viruses. The considerable interest in synthetic vectors for the delivery of nucleic-acid-based vaccines and therapeutics is supported by the following advantages. There is no limit in terms of genetic capacity. Moreover, since there is no immune response against chemical non-viral vectors, repeated administration of the drug is allowed. Finally, ease of manufacturing, lower costs, and process reproducibility for various nucleic acids make them attractive candidates for gene therapy, genome editing, and vaccine development.

## 6.1 Polyplexes

The polyelectrolyte theory states that polyanionic compounds bear an extended shape because of intramolecular anionic repulsion and that in the presence of a polycationic polymer, both polymers will associate, resulting in a compacted state (Figure 6.1).

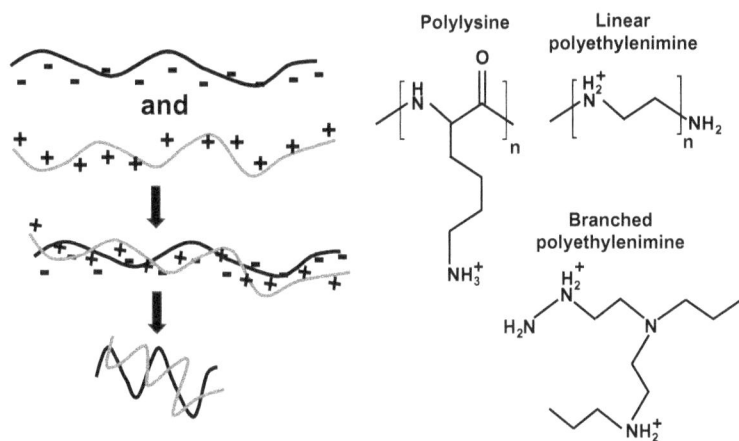

**Figure 6.1.** Polyplex self-formation and condensation, and formulas of the most widely used cationic polymer for DNA or RNA delivery and cell transfection.

The complexes formed by polycationic polymers with nucleotides have been designated as polyplexes. Initially, polylysine was used as the most popular polyplex-forming polycationic polymer. Subsequently, more efficient compounds have been introduced, such as polyethylenei-mine (PEI; Figure 6.1). Polyamidoamine (PAMAM) dendrimers have also been used as synthetic gene delivery vectors.

## 6.2 Lipoplexes

Lipids, carrying a cationic head, self-assemble in water to cationic micelles. When they are mixed with a neutral lipid, they can form a planar, polycationic bilayer. Such a polycationic surface has been shown to form a self-assembling system with olidodeoxyribonucleotides, siRNA, plasmid DNA, or mRNA and to provide a highly versatile generation of non-viral gene delivery vectors.

Hundreds of such lipids have been proposed, whose geometry is schematized in Figure 6.2. Basically, the hydrophobic moiety is composed of a dialkyl or trialkyl moiety, whose length is generally between 14 and 18 carbons per arm. This hydrophobic tail is attached to a cationic head through a neutral linker of variable length and composition. The cationic

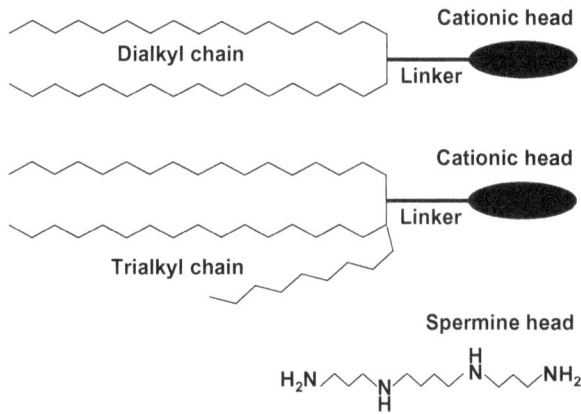

**Figure 6.2.**   Basic structure of cationic lipids used for gene delivery. Cationic charges from the heads are, in most cases, moieties of amines — either quaternary ammonium or tertiary/secondary amines, such as in spermine.

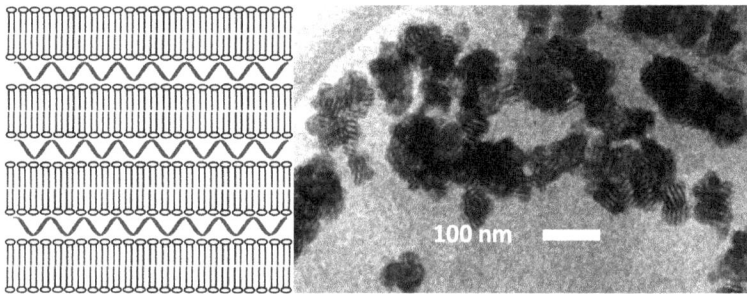

**Figure 6.3.**   Schematic representation and microscopic image of a lipoplex composed of plasmid DNA and a cationic lipid carrying a spermine moiety (negative-staining electron microscopy).

*Source*: Adapted from Pitard *et al.* (1997)

head is generally composed of secondary, tertiary or quaternary amines. The spermine polyamine has been widely used as a cationic head.

X-ray diffraction, electron microscopy, and small-angle light diffraction scattering have been used to characterize lipoplex structure. A periodic organization has been observed, consisting of several lamellae.

Particles of 100–200 nm size (i.e., similar to those of a virus) are evidenced by electron microscopy, where black bands can be attributed to the nucleic acid content, which are interspaced by "white" lipid bilayers. A periodicity of 6.5 nm in the lamellar structure has been determined by X-ray scattering. Because the membrane thickness is 3.9 nm, the thickness of the water layer is 2.6 nm, which is sufficient to include a hydrated DNA double helix with a total diameter of 2.5 nm. The schematized sandwich-like structure, along with an electron microscopy image of a lipoplex obtained through negative staining, is displayed in Figure 6.3.

## 6.3 Physico-Chemistry of Polyplexes and Lipoplexes

The ratio between the vector cationic charges and the polynucleotide phosphate linkage anionic charges is an important formulation factor. Since the vast majority of cationic vectors contain amines, this ratio is often referred to as the N/P ratio. It has been found that a positive N/P ratio is favorable for binding to the cell membrane and further intracellular internalization. A positive N/P net charge ratio of lipoplexes and polyplexes also ensures the colloidal stability of self-assembling nanometer-sized systems because of the electrostatic repulsion between nanoparticles exhibiting a positive surface zeta potential. A negative N/P ratio also ensures colloidal stability; however, negatively charged nanoparticles do not efficiently transfect cells. Finally, an N/P charge ratio of approximately 1 induces massive aggregation of both polyplexes and lipoplexes, as shown in Figure 6.4.

When calculating this charge ratio, care should be taken to the fact that all amines from a cationic polyamine head might not be protonated under cationic state. Indeed, in spermine, for instance, all polyamines are not equivalent, and at pH 7, only about two or three out of four amines are cationic.

In addition, it has been observed that cationic lipoplexes or polyplexes exhibit certain toxicity when used *in vivo*. This is primarily because they are intrinsically toxic to the cells; furthermore, when injected into the bloodstream, they cause red blood cell and platelet aggregation and retention in the lung capillary endothelium. These unwanted inflammatory

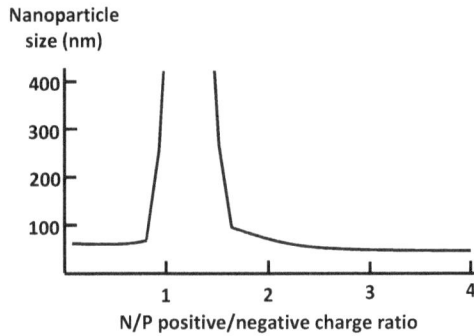

**Figure 6.4.** Physico-chemistry of polyplexes and lipoplexes: importance of the N/P charge ratio on the colloidal stability and particle size.

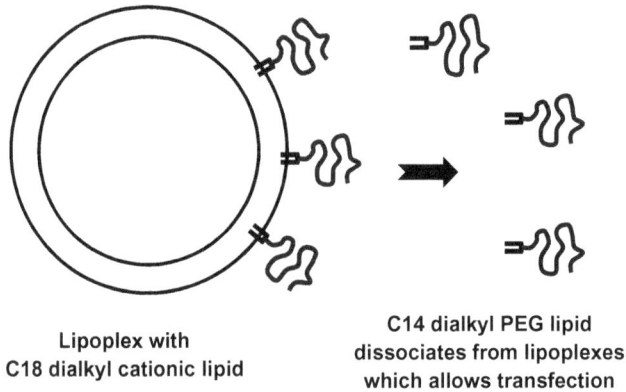

**Figure 6.5.** The PEG lipid shields the lipoplex surface. The dialkyl chain of the PEG lipid is shorter (C14) than that of the cationic lipid (C18). Because of this smaller hydrophobic moiety and the highly hydrophilic PEG, the PEG lipid can dissociate from the lipoplex, thus allowing lipoplex unshielding and efficient transfection.

effects can be circumvented by shielding lipoplexes and polyplexes surfaces with neutral hydrophilic polymers, such as polyethylene glycol. For polyplexes, these polymers can be covalently linked to cationic polymeric vectors. In lipoplexes, lipids carrying a PEG head (usually of 2,000 kDa MW PEG linear polymer) are added to the formulation.

When using PEG shielding components, care should be taken to account for the fact that PEG-induced steric hindrance can potentially prevent lipoplex or polyplex from binding to the target cell membrane and thus inhibit transfection. Thus, PEG shielding should be readily dissociable from the lipoplexes or polyplexes. In lipoplexes, this is obtained by using PEG-lipid with a short dialkyl moiety (C14–C15), which can more easily dissociate from the lipoplexes than di-C18 alkyl chains (Figure 6.5).

## 6.4 Mechanism of DNA and RNA Cellular Uptake

The widely recognized mechanism of DNA and RNA cellular uptake when delivered by chemical vectors is schematized in Figure 6.6. In a first step (Figure 6.6(A)), the cationic polyplex or lipoplex binds to the cell membrane. In the example illustrated in this figure, the negative staining electron microscopy image of a lipoplex is depicted. In a second step, the lipoplex is taken up by the cell through an endocytic mechanism (Figure 6.6(B)). Endosomal breakdown then allows DNA/RNA delivery to the cytosol (Figure 6.6(C); see Sections 6.5 and 6.6).

Once in the cytosol, mRNA, ASO, or siRNA ensure their desired function. If DNA were delivered, for instance in gene replacement therapy, it must gain access to the nucleus, and this is generally impaired by the nuclear envelope. It has been observed that very few, if any, plasmid DNA molecules gain access to the nucleus in post-mitotic, non-dividing cells. During mitosis, the nuclear envelope is disrupted, which allows some plasmid DNA to be sequestered into the nucleus of the daughter cells. This explains why plasmid or large DNA delivery by cationic lipids is

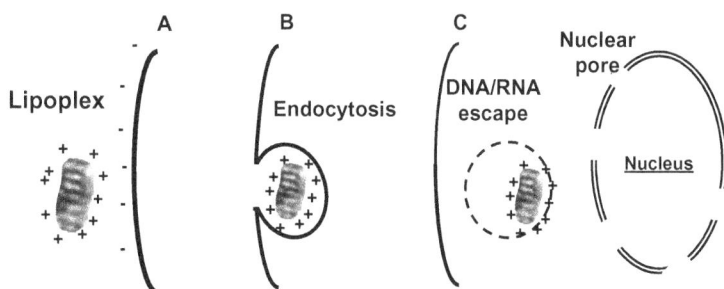

**Figure 6.6.** Mechanism of lipoplexes entry into the cell.

efficient *in vitro* on dividing cells in culture; however, transfection is inefficient *in vivo* on quiescent cells.

## 6.5  Mechanism of DNA/RNA Endosomal Leakage via Membrane Fusion

Several mechanisms have been proposed in order to explain the endosomal breakdown responsible for DNA or RNA delivery to the cytosol. In the first mechanism, it is postulated that the binding and fusion of cationic lipid bilayers with the negatively charged endosomal phospholipid bilayer destabilize this endosomal bilayer and induce endosome leakiness. Lipid bilayer fusion and endosomal membrane destabilization are favored by "cone-shaped" cationic lipids, in which the cross-section of the cationic head is smaller than that of the hydrophobic lipid moiety (Figure 6.7).

According to the molecular shape hypothesis, cone-shaped lipids are incompatible with a bilayer and are more likely to form structures, such as inverted hexagonal phases that can disrupt the endosomal membrane.

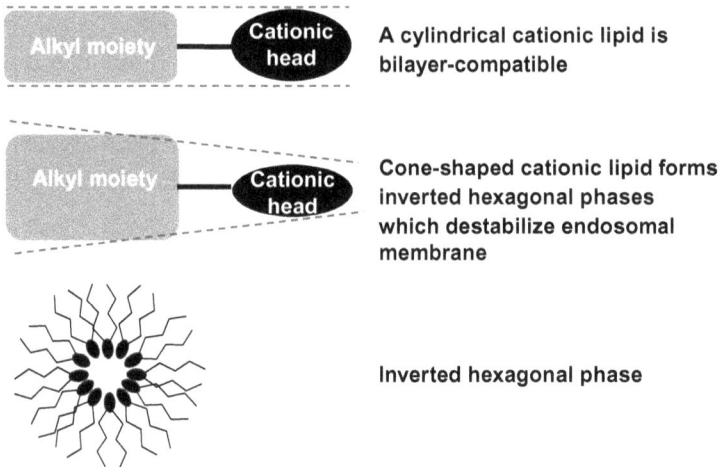

**Figure 6.7.**  Cone-shaped cationic lipid forms inverted hexagonal phases, which are considered to be membrane destabilizing and endosomal disrupting agents.

Hence, cationic lipids containing three or even four alkyl chains are now considered to display the highest endosomolytic activity. The introduction of one or two double bonds in the alkyl chain also allows an increase in the cross-section of the hydrophobic alkyl moiety and the disorganization of the lipidic bilayers while increasing fluidity.

The fusion mechanism has been postulated to account for the transfection efficacy of cationic lipids bearing a quaternary ammonium group, such as 1,2-dioleoyl-3-trimethylammonium propane (DOTAP) and ionizable LNPs (discussed in the following section). The transfectant DOTAP (available as a salt of chloride or methylsulfate) is a widely used first-generation fusogenic cationic lipid, which contains a quaternary ammonium and one carbon-carbon double bond in each alkyk chain. DOTAP is usually associated with the neutral lipid dioleoylphosphatidylethanolamine (DOPE) (Figure 6.8). Figure 6.8 also shows a typical transfection agent carrying a spermine moiety with a cationic head, which has proven to be efficient for transfecting a large variety of cells.

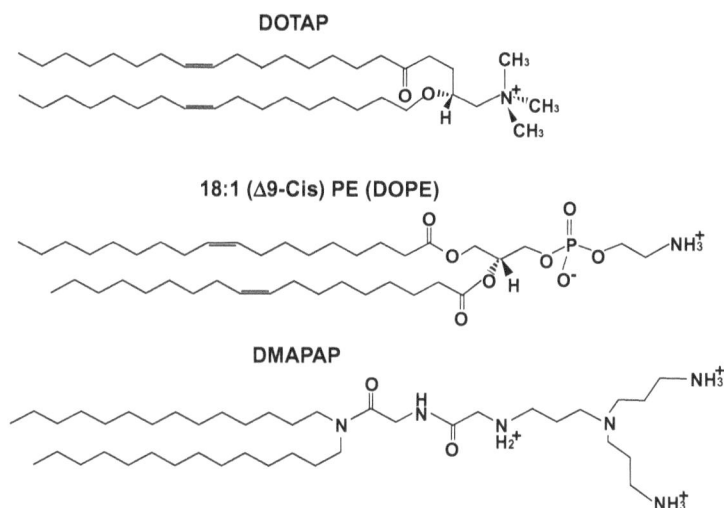

**Figure 6.8.** Chemical structure of the fusogenic cationic lipid DOTAP, the neutral colipid DOPE, or the polyamine carrying a globular head DMAPAP: 2-{3-[Bis-(3-amino-propyl)-amino]-propylamino}-N-ditetradecyl carbamoyl methyl-acetamide.

## 6.6 Mechanism of DNA/RNA Endosomal Leakage by the Proton Pump Hypothesis

The second endosomal escape mechanism is called the "proton sponge effect". It has been introduced in order to explain the high transfection efficacy of cationic vectors containing polyamines, in which the amino groups are incompletely cationized at a physiologically neutral pH. The first generation of such vectors contained either a spermine or sperm-ine analog, such as lipofectamine, or the lipid DMAPAP, as shown in Figure 6.8. This mechanism is based on the action of the proton-pump ATPase, which acidifies endosomes and lysosomes down to a pH of 6 for endosomes and pH between 4.5 and 5 for lysosomes.

The active uptake of protons, mediated by the pump, occurs together with chloride anion uptake to ensure electrical neutrality (Figure 6.9). Because the polymer or lipid transfection agent contains secondary and tertiary amines, some of them unprotonated at a physiological pH of 7, the

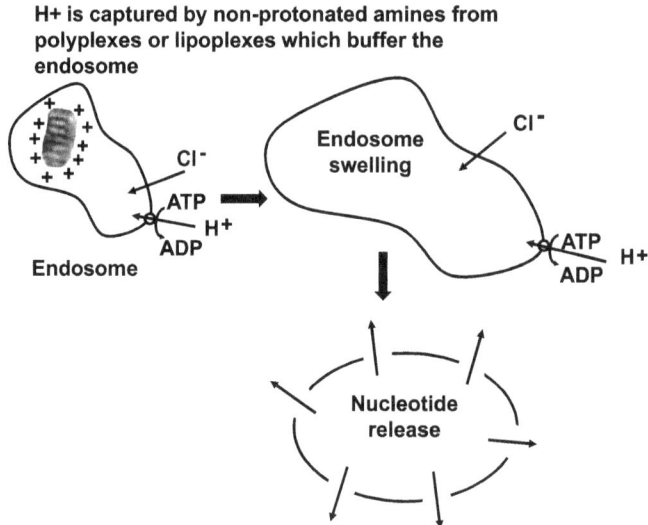

**Figure 6.9.** The proton pump hypothesis for endosomal disruption and nucleotide release to the cytosol. The swelling and leakage of endosomes are caused by an excess of proton and chloride ion transport, which is due to proton complexation with unprotonated amines in the chemical transfection vector, either a cationic polymer or cationic lipid.

protons pumped into the endosome are captured by these amines. This "buffering" capacity induces the sustained uptake by the endolysosomes of a large number of protons and concomitant chloride counterions to equilibrate the electric charges, before the final acidic pH of 5–6 is reached. This increase in intraendosomal $H^+Cl^-$ concentration, in turn, induces water to enter the endolysosomal compartment in order to equilibrate osmolarity. The resultant swelling of the endolysosomal compartment leads to membrane destabilization and breakdown. This effect has been coined the "proton sponge" effect because the unprotonated amine of the vector complexes protons like a sponge. It has been proposed to account for the transfection efficacy of both lipids containing unprotonated amines at a pH of 7 and PEI, in which the high density of amine groups leads to about 30% of them being unprotonated at that pH.

The exact process leading to the cytosolic release of the genetic drugs from the endolysosomal compartment might result from a combination of both membrane destabilization and fusion, as described in Section 6.5, together with the proton sponge effect.

## 6.7 LNPs Containing Ionizable Cationic Lipids

The most recent advancement in self-assembling systems for RNA or DNA delivery involves LNPs, which have gained widespread recognition and use since their clinical approval for the treatment of certain genetic disorders and for mRNA vaccines. The first clinical use has been for treating the rare disease, transthyretin amyloidosis, with siRNA *patisiran* (Onpattro) administered IV, which targets the liver. Following this historical breakthrough, two LNP mRNA vaccines against COVID-19 were subsequently granted clinical approval as LNP drugs: Comirnaty and Spikevax. Hundreds of millions of doses of these two drugs have been administered as intramuscular mRNA vaccines.

The notable LNP feature is the presence of an "ionizable" lipid, usually a tertiary amine, displaying a pKa ranging from 5.5 to 6.5. Although this requirement was established by an *in vivo* screen of a large number of different lipids for Factor IX mRNA silencing in the liver, early works had already identified the usefulness of ionizable amines for transfection vectors, for instance in PEI, spermine-bearing lipids, or lipids equipped with a histidine ionizable moiety. The LNP rationale is that lipids with a pKa in the moderate range of 5.5–6.5 can be fully charged at a pH of 5, allowing self-complexation with DNA or RNA molecules. The resulting lipoplex can then be titrated until reaching a neutral zeta surface potential at a physiological pH of 7, thus allowing biocompatible *in vivo* administration and avoiding disruption by blood anionic components, such as albumin. Finally, another advantage is that LNPs become cationic again in the acidic endolysosomal compartments, thus leading to fusion with the endolysosomal membrane, to endolysosomal disruption, and to DNA or RNA payload delivery to the cell cytosol through the two mechanisms described above: the fusogenic activity of trialkyl-bearing cationic lipids and the proton sponge effect.

The LNP formulation which has been selected for patisiran includes buffer components (disodium hydrogen phosphate, heptahydrate potassium dihydrogen phosphate, and anhydrous sodium chloride), as well as the lipid DLin-MC3-DMA ((6Z,9Z,28Z,31Z)-heptatriaconta-6,9,28,31-tetraen-19-yl-4-(dimethylamino) butanoate), an amine-containing ionizable lipid with a pKa of 6.4 (Figure 6.10). In addition, the formulation comprises the neutral lipid distearoylphosphatidylcholine, cholesterol, and the PEGylated lipid DMG-PEG 2000 (Figure 6.11(A)). Each 1 mL of Onpattro also contains 6.2 mg of cholesterol USP, 13.0 mg of DLin-MC3-DMA, 3.3 mg of disteroylphosphatidylcholine DSPC, and 1.6 mg of α-(3'-{[1,2-di(myristyloxy)propanoxy] carbonylamino} propyl)-.-methoxy, polyoxyethylene) designed as PEG2000 C-DMG.

In such a typical LNP formulation, cholesterol is added to provide rigidity to the 40–100 nm nanoparticles. The neutral lipid distearoylphosphatidylcholine attenuates the charge repulsion between the DLin-MC3-DMA cationic heads. In addition, the PEGylated lipid PEG2000 C-DMG ensures colloidal stability through the highly hydrated polyethyleneglycol chains forming a protective shield around the nanoparticle.

The structure of the ionizable lipid of each of the three clinically approved formulations is displayed in Figure 6.10. Each exhibits a tertiary

**DLin-MC3-DMA — Component of Onpattro siRNA LNP drug**
Z,28Z,31Z)-Heptatriaconta-6,9,28,31-tetraen-19-yl 4-(dimethylamino)butanoate

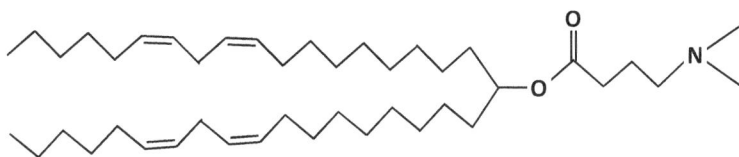

**ALC-0315 — Component of Comirnaty mRNA vaccine**
6-((2-hexyldecanoyl)oxy)-N-(6-((2-hexyldecanoyl)oxy)hexyl)-N-(4-hydroxybutyl) hexan-1-aminium

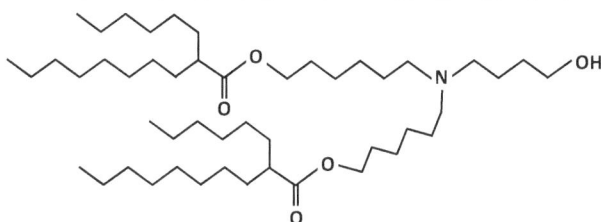

**SM-102 — Component of Spikevax mRNA vaccine**
1-octylnonyl 8-[(2-hydroxyethyl)[6-oxo-6- (undecyloxy)hexyl]amino]- octanoate

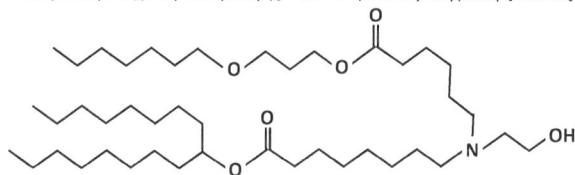

**Figure 6.10.** The three ionizable lipid components of clinically approved formulations for the siRNA drug patisiran against transthyretin amyloidosis and for the mRNA vaccines Comirnaty and Spikevax against COVID-19.

amine with a slightly acidic pKa, thus being unprotonated at physiological pH 7 and allowing intra-endosomal protonation. The unsaturated double bonds in DLin-MC3-DMA were introduced in order to enhance endo-somal membrane destabilization and disruption through the formation of a non-bilayer phase. The hydrophobic moiety of DLin-MC3-DMA is composed of dilinoleic alkyl tail, raising concerns regarding its chronic use because of potential accumulation and toxicity, particularly in the liver. Hence, the mRNA vaccine lipids ALC-0315 and SM-102 contain several ester linkages, with the aim of increasing their biodegradability through the action of endogenous esterases. Moreover, the multibranched

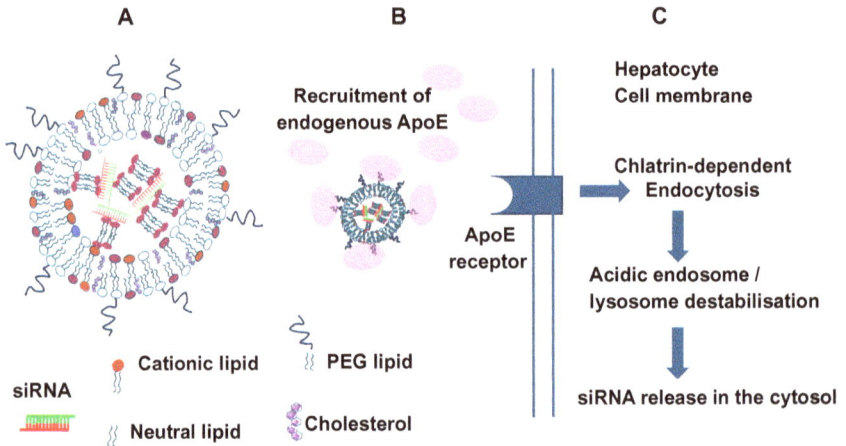

**Figure 6.11.** (A) siRNAs encapsulated in LNPs are protected from the actions of nucleases and targeted to liver. LNPs are specifically targeted to the liver because they bind apolipoproteins E (ApoE proteins) in the blood circulation and then bind to the ApoE-LDL receptor on the hepatocyte surface. (B) LNP decorated with Apo E bind to ApoE receptor on the hepatocyte plasma membrane. (C) DLin-MC3-DMA lipids at the LNP surface are neutral at a pH of 7. Inside the endosome, DLin-MC3-DMA becomes cationic, which favors either fusion with the endosome membrane and siRNA release or endosome breakdown caused by the "proton pump" osmotic effect. The figure represents a siRNA LNP, but it is also valid for mRNA LNPs.

geometry of ALC-0315 and SM-102 increases their cone-shape property and hence their fusogenicity.

In addition to their protective effect against RNase or DNase attributed to the polyethyleneglycol shield, as well as their endolysosome disruption capacity, LNPs also show an advantageous capacity for near-exclusive delivery to the liver when they are injected intravenously. It has long been known that some colloidal delivery systems, such as nanoparticles or liposomes, accumulate rapidly in the liver and spleen upon IV administration, in a proportion superior to 90%. Nanoparticles or liposomes containing ionizable lipids thus represent an inherently favorable system for high-yield encapsulation of negatively charged siRNA or mRNA and for preferential liver uptake, as already previously demonstrated for DNA. Initial assumption was that uptake by Kupfer cells of the reticulo-endothelial system was responsible for the high level of LNPs capture by liver.

However, a more complex mechanism has been evidenced recently, which can account for the delivery of DNA/RNA payload to hepatocytes.

The mechanism by which the LNPs are targeted at the liver hepatocytes is schematized in Figure 6.11. It involves the natural binding of the plasma protein ApoE to the PEGylated LNPs. Since liver hepatocytes express a high concentration of the ApoE receptor, LNPs decorated with ApoE bind to hepatocyte cell membranes. The resulting ApoE receptor clustering induces internalization through a clathrin-dependent endocytosis mechanism.

By binding to the LNP surface, ApoE proteins form a so-called "corona". The composition of the corona depends on each LNP formulation, which will determine its ultimate fate in the body after IV administration. It has been demonstrated that ApoE is the major component of the corona of PEG-lipid-containing LNPs, thus leading to liver gene delivery through an endogenous targeting process.

Inside the endosome, it is postulated that the ionizable DLin-MC3-DMA lipid becomes cationic because of the endosomal/lysosomal acidification. This induces endosome breakdown, for which two different mechanisms have been proposed (Sections 6.5 and 6.6):

(1) In the first one, the ionizable DLin-MC3-DMA lipid on the LNP surface becomes cationic within the acidic endosomal compartment, leading to the fusion of the positively charged LNP surface with the negatively charged endosome membrane.

(2) According to the alternative proton-sponge mechanism detailed above, the ionizable lipid captures and titrates the $H^+$ ions that are taken up into the endosomes by the endolysosomal proton-pump ATPase. This induces the sustained uptake of a large number of protons and chloride anions, which diffuse into the endosomes to equilibrate the proton cationic charge. This proton sponge effect induces water entry, which in turn induces endosome swelling and breakdown.

Both postulated mechanisms result in siRNA release into the cytosol and further interaction with the RNA-induced silencing complex (RISC; see Section 6.8). *Patisiran* was granted orphan drug status, fast-track designation, priority review, and breakthrough therapy designation due to its

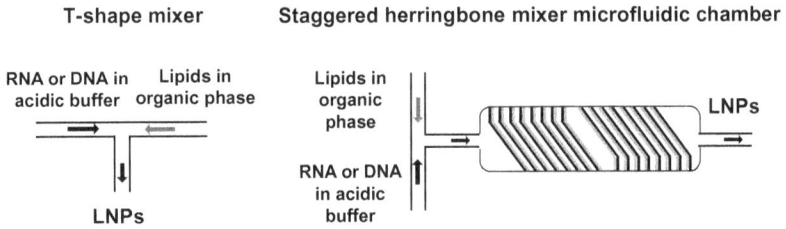

**Figure 6.12.**    Scheme diagram of two technologies for preparing homogeneous populations of LNPs. On the right-and side, a microfluidic device is depicted.

novel mechanism and the rarity of the condition it treats. It has been approved for medical use in the USA and the EU in August 2018. Since then, LNP use as mRNA delivery vectors has grown exponentially for two types of applications: (1) vaccines by delivering mRNA encoding viral proteins, and (2) gene-, base-, or prime-editing applications by delivering mRNA encoding CRISPR-Cas9 and its variants, together with the RNA guide (see Chapter 9).

Identifying ways to produce large amounts of LNPs in a reproducible manner has shown great progress in recent years. Typically, nucleic acids in acidic aqueous buffers are rapidly mixed with the lipids in the organic phase. This occurs either in a T-shaped mixer or in a microfluidic system equipped, for instance, with a staggered herringbone mixer geometry (Figure 6.12).

## 6.8   Targeting Hepatocytes via the Asialoglycoprotein Receptor

The accelerating pace of science is brightly illustrated by the fact that, only a few years after the clinical approval of LNPs for siRNA delivery to the liver, a new technology appeared, which is based on the principle of sugar functionalization to target the hepatocyte asialoglycoprotein receptor (ASGPR) and which has rapidly become the preferred approach for siRNA delivery to the liver. However, this strategy, which is described in this section, is not the favored technology for mRNA delivery to the liver, for which PEG-covered LNPs remain the most potent delivery vectors.

The biological function of ASPGR involves capturing degraded proteins from the blood circulation. Circulating proteins are all glycoproteins possessing a N-acetyl neuraminic acid residue, which is also called sialic acids and constitutes the terminal sugar of their glycosidic moiety. Proper sialylation is a critical signal indicating that a protein circulating in the blood or present at the cell surface can perform its biological function. When the sialyl is lost, galactose or N-acetyl galactose amine residues are revealed at the surface of degraded proteins. They are then captured by the ASGPR and taken up into hepatocytes for degradation of such unproper proteins.

The ASGPR is thus a lectin which specifically binds to galactose or N-acetyl galactose. It is present at a remarkably high density on the hepatocyte surface. There are approximately 500,000 ASGPRs per cell. As shown in Figure 6.13, binding to the ASGPR actively promotes the cellular uptake of the ligand upon clustering and aggregation of several receptors in coated pits. The ASGPR turnover is rapid since only about

## Tri-antennary galactose / ASPGR mediated delivery to hepatocytes

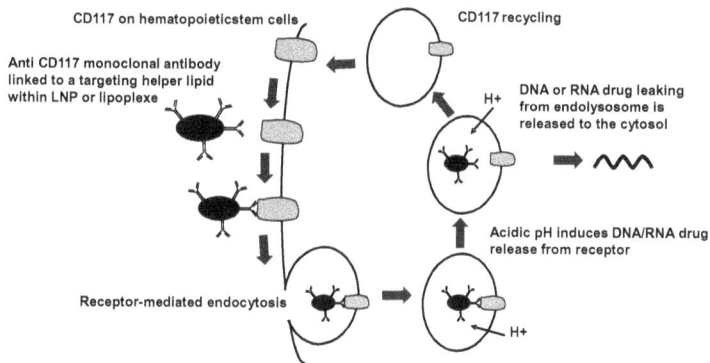

**Figure 6.13.** Schematic representation of genetic drug delivery to hepatocytes. Binding to the ASGPR actively promotes the cellular uptake of the ligand upon clustering and aggregation of several receptors into coated pits. After endocytosis, ASGPR recycling occurs within approximately 15 min concomitantly with the release of the bound ligand in the acidified endosomal compartment. The ASGPR affinity for one galactose or N-acetylglucosamine is in the millimolar range. Since the ASGPR possesses three sugar-binding sites, a tri-antennary ligand presenting three galactose or galactosamine moieties will display an avidity in the nanomolar range. A similar targeting can be achieved using LNPs by adding a helper lipid equipped with three galactose heads or galactosamine moieties or with a poly-galactosylated cationic polymer.

5–10% of ASGPRs are permanently accessible at the cell plasma membrane. After endocytosis, ASGPR recycling occurs within approximately 15 min concomitantly with the release of the bound ligand in the acidified endosomal compartment through a process similar to that of the transferrin receptor cycle. The ASGPR affinity for one galactose or N-acetylglucosamine is in the millimolar range. Since the ASGPR possesses three sugar-binding sites, a tri-antennary ligand with three sugar moieties exhibits nanomolar-range "avidity" resulting from the cooperative affinity of three ligands. Hence, a high ASGPR density on hepatocyte surfaces and fast turnover indicate that this lectin is an ideal candidate for a liver-targeted RNA drug. The fact that more than 80% of an IV-injected compound functionalized by several galactose or galactosamine is taken up by the liver has been evidenced by SPECT or fluorescent *in vivo* imaging techniques using lactosylated albumin.

The first evidence for the potential of a targeting ligand bearing three-sugar moiety for gene delivery to the liver was obtained in 1987 through *in vitro* experiments, coupling the protein asialoorosomucoid with polylysine. Following this, several lipids bearing a tri-antennary galactosyl residue were synthesized. When added to a conventional lipoplex, an increase of up to 1,000-fold in gene delivery can be observed. This large increase in transfection efficiency was further confirmed by grafting galactosyl residues onto other transfection polymers, such as polyethyleneimine.

The clinical realization of this strategy has been established through the covalent linkage of a tri-antennary N-aceylgalactosamine triGalNac to small interfering RNAs (siRNAs; see Chapter 11 on siRNA mechanism and examples of application). The principle involves the functionalization of the sense passenger strand with high-affinity/-avidity ASGPR-targeting moiety, carrying three N-acetyl-galactosamine residues (triGalNac).

As shown in Figure 6.14, the tri-GalNac is covalently linked to the 3' end of the siRNA sense strand, thus ensuring the absence of effect on the binding of its complementary antisense to RISC which is responsible of the silecing effect. The cellular delivery mechanism is schematized in Figure 6.15 (see Chapter 11 for more details on the siRNA action mechanism).

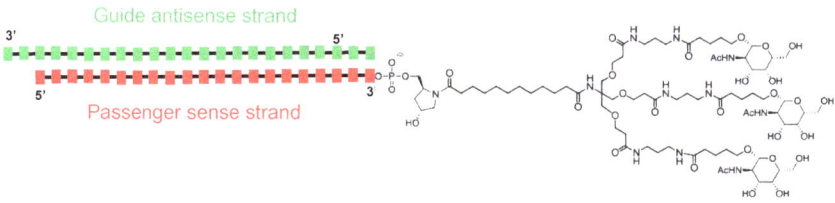

**Figure 6.14.** Tri-GalNac chemical group addressing siRNA to the hepatocyte ASGPR. The tri-GalNac is covalently linked to the 3' end of the siRNA sense strand, thus ensuring the absence of effect on the capture by RISC of the complementary antisense strand necessary for mRNA cleavage.

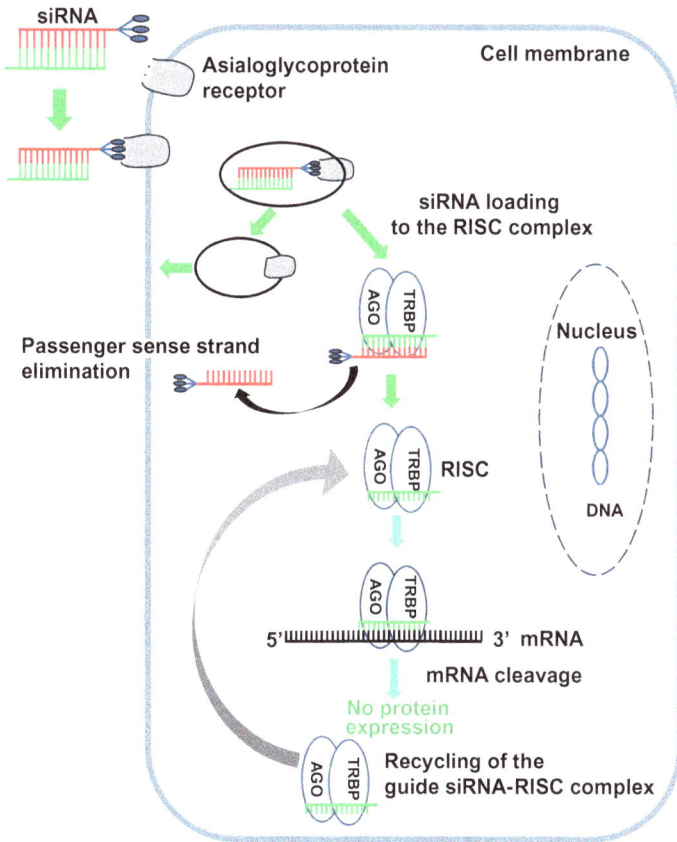

**Figure 6.15.** Mechanism of siRNA delivery to liver hepatocytes by targeting the ASGPR.

The first clinically approved drug of that family is *vutrisiran*, an siRNA against transthyretin for the treatment of transthyretin amyloidosis. The improved metabolic stability of *vutrisiran* and the highly potent targeting efficacy of its tri-Gal-Nac lead to an exceptional intrinsic efficacy. This is demonstrated by the therapeutic efficacy of very low doses and the exceptionally long duration of action, since an administration every three months is sufficient to achieve a similar therapeutic effect as *patisiran*, the LNP siRNA developed against the same genetic disease. Polyneuropathy, cardiomyopathy, and wild-type transthyretin amyloidosis are all envisioned as *vutrisiran* indications.

## 6.9 Diverse LNP Targeting Strategies

An increasing number of targeting strategies have been proposed. For instance, other cell types express specific sugar receptors, such as liver Kupffer cells and liver sinusoidal endothelial cells which express a mannose receptor and are involved in adaptive and innate immunity through their antigen-presenting capacity. Poly-histidine transfecting vectors functionalized with mannose residues have been described. They target mannose receptors (MRs) and DC-specific intercellular adhesion molecule-3-grabbing non-integrin (DC-SIGN) receptors. The MRs (CD206) and DC-SIGN receptors (CD209) induce a clathrin-dependent mediated endocytosis of high-mannose oligosaccharides in dendritic cells. These cells are the main antigen-presenting cells, and they induce cytotoxic CD8+ T lymphocytes against the antigen. The MRs are expressed not only in dendritic cells but also in various other cell types, including monocytes, macrophages (including liver Kupffer cells), and subsets of endothelial and epithelial cells. In contrast, DC-SIGN receptors are only expressed by dendritic cells. Polymannosylated LNPs or cationic polymers are considered of interest for cancer treatment, through the transfection of genes encoding tumor-specific antigens.

As other examples, a peptide binding to specific integrins would have the capacity to target inflammatory endothelium, or functionalizing an LNP or lipoplex with a hormone would target the extracellular hormone receptor, such as insulin for hepatocyte targeting. Transferrin has also been proposed as an interesting targeting head because of the high density of transferrin receptors on tumor cells and brain capillaries. Gene delivery to the brain is an important and mainly unsolved challenge, and transferrin receptor-binding peptides are considered potentially valuable, given the claimed capacity of the transferrin receptor of brain capillary endothelial cells to undergo transcytosis and release its cargo to the brain parenchyma.

Attempts concerning immunolipoplexes equipped with a monoclonal antibody are numerous, for instance, an antibody targeting prostate-specific membrane antigen (PSMA) for delivering anticancer genetic drugs to the prostate. In another example, mRNA-LNPs were conjugated with antibodies (Abs) specific to the vascular cell adhesion molecule, PECAM-1, leading to strong inhibition of hepatic uptake after IV injection, concomitantly with approximatively 200-fold elevation of mRNA delivery and 25-fold increase in protein expression in the lungs, as compared to non-targeted counterparts. Unlike hepatic delivery of LNP-mRNA, Ab-LNP-mRNA is independent of ApoE. Vascular re-targeting of mRNA represents a promising, powerful, and unique approach for novel experimental and clinical interventions in organs of interest other than liver.

Exciting prospects concern the delivery of genome editing mRNA (Chapter 9) using immune-targeted liposomes. For instance, hematopoietic stem cells (HSCs), which are the source of all blood cells, can be modified *in vivo* with high efficacy by using mRNA-LNPs conjugated with an anti-CD117 monoclonal antibody (Figure 6.16). In 2024, it was reported that the delivery of the anti-human CD117/LNP-based editing system yielded near-complete correction of the mutation in the hemoglobin $\beta$ subunit in hematopoietic sickle cells. Depletion of HSCs could also be achieved through similar targeted LNP delivery of a pro-apoptotic mRNA.

An interesting indirect mechanism has been proposed to explain the targeting of pulmonary endothelium by cationic LNPs: in blood circulation, cationic LNPs are covered by a serum protein corona characterized by a relatively high content of vitronectin. This contrasts with PEG-covered LNPs, which preferentially bind ApoE (see the previous section).

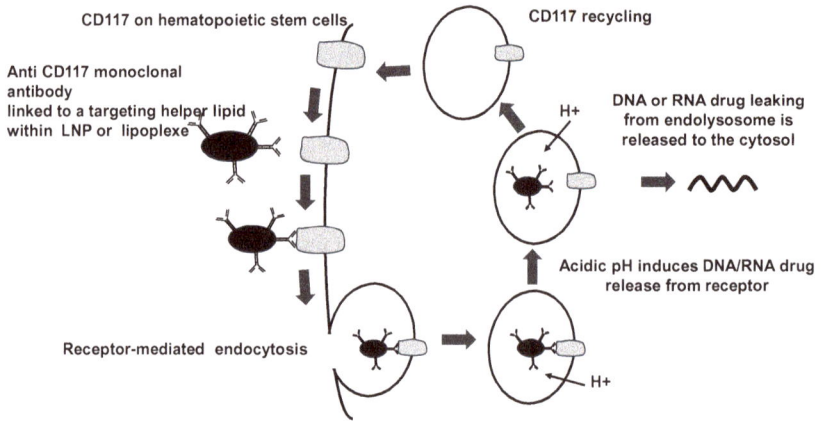

**Figure 6.16.**   Targeting of LNPs to HSCs using a monoclonal antibody against the CD117 surface marker.

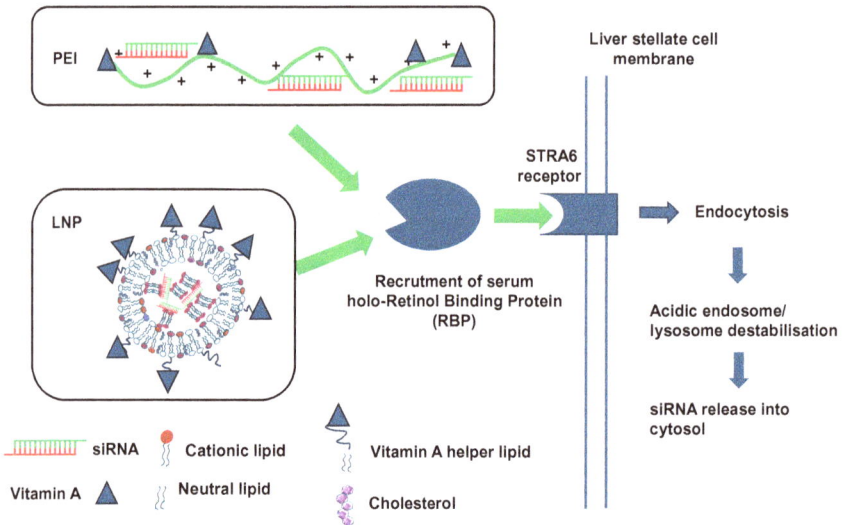

**Figure 6.17.**   Retinol (vitamin A)-mediated targeting of PEI or LNPs to hepatic stellate cells or other fibrotic cells harboring the STRA6 receptor. In the figure, LNP or PEI are represented for siRNA delivery as an example, however, the strategy is also valid for mRNA or DNA delivery.

Subsequently, vitronectin's affinity for lung endothelium ensures efficient LNP targeting to the lung.

A mechanism specifically involving another serum protein is worth mentioning here as a strategy which could be generalized to other systems. The receptor STRA6 is a transmembrane cell-surface receptor of the blood-circulating retinol-binding protein. This receptor is responsible for the transport of retinol (a type of vitamin A) to specific sites, such as the eye or liver stellate cells. This occurs through the removal of retinol from the blood-borne holo-Retinol Binding Protein (RBP) and transport into the cell, where it is metabolized into retinoic acid. It has been shown that LNPs containing an "helper" lipid carrying vitamin A, or PEI conjugated with vitamin A as the targeting head, were able to deliver siRNA drugs to hepatic stellate cells. This presumably occurs through the recruitment of the serum holo-RBP (Figure 6.17). This targeting option is of importance, given the profibrotic action of hepatic stellate cells, because it has the potential to inhibit the synthesis of fibrotic components such as collagen by delivering an siRNA against a collagen chaperone protein. This approach has also been proposed for the treatment of pancreatic and lung fibrosis.

## Bibliography

Behr JP. Synthetic gene transfer vectors II: back to the future. *Acc Chem Res*. 2012 Jul;45(7):980–4. doi: 10.1021/ar200213g.

Billingsley MM, Gong N, Mukalel AJ, Thatte AS, El-Mayta R, Patel SK, Metzloff AE, Swingle KL, et al. *In vivo* mRNA CAR T cell engineering via targeted ionizable lipid nanoparticles with extrahepatic tropism. *Small*. 2024 Mar;20(11):e2304378. doi: 10.1002/smll.202304378.

Boussif O, Lezoualc'h F, Zanta MA, Mergny MD, Scherman D, Demeneix B, Behr JP. A versatile vector for gene and oligonucleotide transfer into cells in culture and *in vivo*: polyethylenimine. *Proc Natl Acad Sci U S A*. 1995 Aug;92(16):7297–301. doi: 10.1073/pnas.92.16.7297.

Breda L, Papp TE, Triebwasser MP, Yadegari A, Fedorky MT, Tanaka N, Abdulmalik O, Pavani G, et al. *In vivo* hematopoietic stem cell modification by mRNA delivery. *Science*. 2023 Jul;381(6656):436–443. doi: 10.1126/science.ade6967.

Byk G, Dubertret C, Escriou V, Frederic M, Jaslin G, Rangara R, Pitard B, Crouzet J, Wils P, Schwartz B, Scherman D. Synthesis, activity, and structure-activity relationship studies of novel cationic lipids for DNA transfer. *J Med Chem*. 1998 Jan;41(2):229–35. doi: 10.1021/jm9704964.

Chaumet-Riffaud P, Martinez-Duncker I, Marty AL, Richard C, Prigent A, Moati F, Sarda-Mantel L, Scherman D, *et al*. Synthesis and application of lactosylated, 99mTc chelating albumin for measurement of liver function. *Bioconjug Chem*. 2010 Apr;21(4):589–96. doi: 10.1021/bc900275f.

Cullis PR, Felgner PL. The 60-year evolution of lipid nanoparticles for nucleic acid delivery. *Nat Rev Drug Discov*. 2024 Jul;4. doi: 10.1038/s41573-024-00977-6.

Escriou V, Ciolina C, Helbling-Leclerc A, Wils P, Scherman D. Cationic lipid-mediated gene transfer: analysis of cellular uptake and nuclear import of plasmid DNA. *Cell Biol Toxicol*. 1998;14(2):95–104.

Gao H, Gonçalves C, Gallego T, François-Heude M, Malard V, Mateo V, Lemoine F, Cendret V, *et al*. Comparative binding and uptake of liposomes decorated with mannose oligosaccharides by cells expressing the mannose receptor or DC-SIGN. *Carbohydr Res*. 2020 Jan;487:107877. doi: 10.1016/j.carres.2019.107877.

Han X, Gong N, Xue L, Billingsley MM, El-Mayta R, Shepherd SJ, Alameh MG, Weissman D, Mitchell MJ. Ligand-tethered lipid nanoparticles for targeted RNA delivery to treat liver fibrosis. *Nat Commun*. 2023 Jan;14(1):75. doi: 10.1038/s41467-022-35637-z.

Parhiz H, Shuvaev VV, Pardi N, Khoshnejad M, Kiseleva RY, Brenner JS, Uhler T, Tuyishime S, *et al*. PECAM-1 directed re-targeting of exogenous mRNA providing two orders of magnitude enhancement of vascular delivery and expression in lungs independent of apolipoprotein E-mediated uptake. *J Control Release*. 2018 Dec;291:106–115. doi: 10.1016/j.jconrel.2018.10.015.

Parhiz H, Shuvaev VV, Li Q, Papp TE, Akyianu AA, Shi R, Yadegari A, Shahnawaz H, *et al*. Physiologically based modeling of LNP-mediated delivery of mRNA in the vascular system. *Mol Ther Nucleic Acids*. 2024 Mar;35(2):102175. doi: 10.1016/j.omtn.2024.102175.

Pitard B, Aguerre O, Airiau M, Lachagès AM, Boukhnikachvili T, Byk G, Dubertret C, Herviou C, Scherman D, Mayaux JF, Crouzet J. Virus-sized self-assembling lamellar complexes between plasmid DNA and cationic micelles promote gene transfer. *Proc Natl Acad Sci U S A*. 1997 Dec;94(26):14412–7. doi: 10.1073/pnas.94.26.14412.

Scherman D, Bessodes M, Cameron B, *et al.* Application of lipids and plasmid design for gene delivery to mammalian cells. *Curr Opin Biotechnol*. 1998 Oct;9(5):480–5. doi: 10.1016/s0958-1669(98)80033-5.

Shepherd SJ, Han X, Mukalel AJ, El-Mayta R, Thatte AS, Wu J, Padilla MS, Alameh MG, *et al.* Throughput-scalable manufacturing of SARS-CoV-2 mRNA lipid nanoparticle vaccines. *Proc Natl Acad Sci U S A*. 2023 Aug;120(33):e2303567120. doi: 10.1073/pnas.2303567120.

Tong Wu, Yu Qi, Chen Xu, Dandan Sui, Fu-Jian Xu. HSC-targeted delivery of shRNA-TGF$\beta$1 by vitamin A-functionalized polyaminoglycoside for hepatic fibrosis therapy. *Nano Today*. 2023;50:101887. doi: 10.1016/j.nantod.2023.101887.

Tros de Ilarduya C, Sun Y, Düzgüneş N. Gene delivery by lipoplexes and polyplexes. *Eur J Pharm Sci*. 2010 Jun;40(3):159–70. doi: 10.1016/j.ejps.2010.03.019.

Vaidya A, Moore S, Chatterjee S, Guerrero E, Kim M, Farbiak L, Dilliard SA, Siegwart DJ. Expanding RNAi to kidneys, lungs, and spleen via selective ORgan targeting (SORT) siRNA lipid nanoparticles. *Adv Mater*. 2024 Aug;36(35):e2313791. doi: 10.1002/adma.202313791.

# Chapter 7

# Physical Delivery of Non-Viral Vectors

Efficient and safe *in vivo* plasmid DNA delivery opens attractive perspectives for gene therapy or for gene functional studies. *In vitro* gene transfer of plasmid DNA has been essentially solved by means of cationic lipid or polymer transfection, or through calcium phosphate precipitation. In contrast, efficient *in vivo* non-viral DNA gene transfer appears much more challenging since each delivery system has its own drawbacks and limitations. While viral vectors present higher cell transduction efficiency, non-viral methods using plasmids remain attractive for a variety of reasons: they are easier and cheaper to produce and manage, and they have no transgene insert size limitations. In addition, unlike viral vectors, plasmid DNA does not directly stimulate the acquired immune system, allowing for periodic readministration of non-viral gene therapy or genetic vaccine treatments.

As indicated in Chapter 6, non-viral chemical vectors have little if any ability to deliver large nucleotides to the cell nucleus because of the nuclear envelope barrier. This does not represent any concern for mRNA or small interfering RNA (siRNA), which only need to access the cytosol, nor for antisense oligonucleotides (ASO), because their small size allows them to diffuse through nuclear pores. In contrast, plasmid DNA has been shown to necessitate a mitosis step for reaching the cell nucleus when delivered by a chemical vector. Successful attempts have been made to identify delivery methods using physical forces in order to overcome this

117

bottleneck and deliver large DNA fragments to the nucleus of resting or slowly dividing cells.

All physical techniques which have been proposed to date consist of inducing transient permeabilization of the cell membrane in order to allow nucleic acids to enter the cells. These different techniques have proven useful and convenient for loco-regional gene delivery and are primarily used as convenient and efficient experimental tools for expressing trans-genes in small animals for research and proof-of-concept gene therapy studies. A combination of several of these techniques has been proposed in some cases, for instance, sonoporation-assisted hydrodynamic delivery. Several clinical applications are in development, and techniques such as electrotransfer are also of general use for *in vitro* transfection of certain cell types such as T-lymphocytes. However, currently, most gene replace-ment clinical applications use viral vectors.

## 7.1  Electrotransfer/Electrogene Transfer: Principle and Mechanism

Among the variety of non-viral delivery methods currently under investi-gation, DNA or mRNA electrotransfer *in vivo*, or *in vitro* on non-dividing cells such as lymphocytes, has proven to be one of the most efficient techniques. Several other terms have been used to designate the same technique, including "electrotransfection," "DNA electroporation," and "electrogene therapy." This technology is based on plasmid DNA or mRNA injection into a tissue or a cell suspension, followed by the applica-tion of a defined set of electric pulses to induce DNA or mRNA cellular entry. Electropermeabilization has initially been used to introduce small molecules or nucleic acids into prokaryotic and eukaryotic cells first *in vitro*, then subsequently *in vivo*. A surprisingly high efficiency of plasmid transfection *in vivo* was observed in muscle tissue. A schematic diagram representing the experimental setup for plasmid delivery into small animal muscle is displayed in Figure 7.1. While noninvasive external plate elec-trodes, together with an electroconductive gel (an electrolyte), are used in this example, most *in vivo* applications use invading needle electrodes in

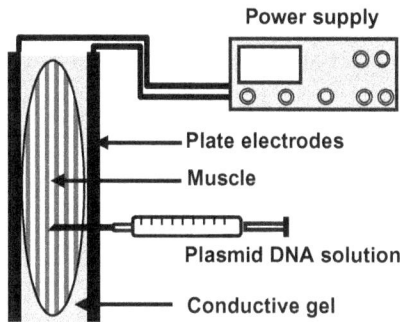

**Figure 7.1.** Experimental setup of a plasmid or mRNA electrotransfer to mouse muscle. The leg muscle is inserted between two plate electrodes, which are connected to a pulse generator. A conductive gel ensures the conduction of electric pulses from the electrodes to the skin. Plasmid DNA is delivered followed by the administration of finely tuned, microsecond or millisecond electric pulses.

order to deliver the DNA/mRNA into a precise and localized region or tissue, for instance for the treatment of brain tumors or in the skin for vaccination purpose.

Electrotransfer can be applied to almost any tissue in a living animal and potentially in humans, including skeletal or smooth muscle, tumors, skin, liver, kidney, arteries, retina, cornea, or even the brain. Skeletal muscle has been the primary tissue chosen for therapeutic and vaccination purposes; however, several investigators have also explored the advantages of delivering to tumors. The efficiency of this electroporation approach has led to clinical trials in the field of DNA immunization or immunotherapy against infectious diseases and cancer.

Figure 7.2 represents the different types of electric pulses that can be delivered by commercial electropulsators. Exponential pulses are often used for *in vitro* transfection, with a time constant dependent on the resistance of the incubation medium. Unipolar square-wave electric pulses are preferred for *in vivo* experiments since the voltage and duration of the pulses can be independently set from the electrical resistance of the tissue. Square-wave bipolar pulses are rather used for electrophysiology, even if they have proven to be efficient for electrotransfer.

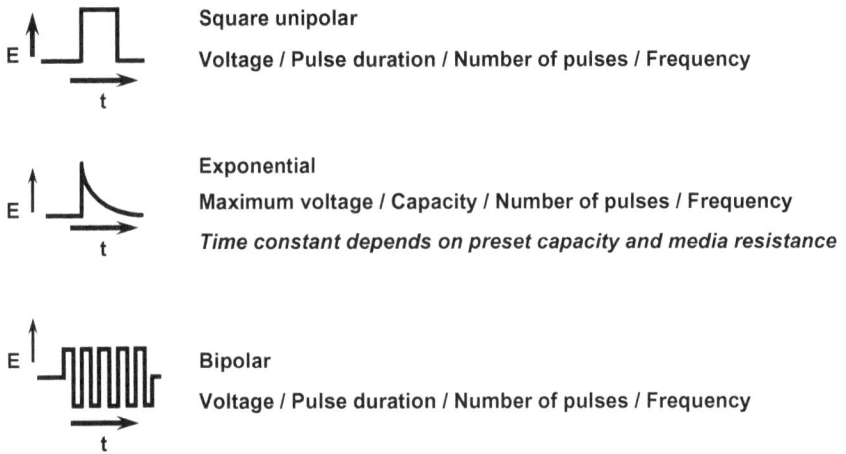

**Figure 7.2.**    Different types of electric pulses used for electrotransfer protocols.

When a cell is submitted to an external electric field, because of the ionic conductance of the intracellular and extracellular medium, which are separated by the non-conducting cellular membrane, a surface charge density is observed at the cell membrane (Figure 7.3). The internal intracellular ionic charge density is negative on the anode side of the cell and positive on the cathode side of the cell. The intracellular charge density has its maximum absolute value at sites where the membrane is perpendicular to the external electric field, and it is null where the cell membrane is parallel to this field.

The ionic charge density at the cell membrane induces a transmembrane potential $\Delta V_m$, whose value depends on the strength of the electric field $E_{ext}$ and the angle $q$ between the electric field and the axis perpendicular to the cell membrane:

$$\Delta V_m = E_{ext} \ 1.5 \ r \cos q \ (Laplace \ law).$$

When $\Delta Vm$ is greater than approximately 0.2 V, this transmembrane potential causes disorganization of the biological phospholipid bilayer and its concomitant permeabilization.

It has to be noted that this transmembrane potential is additive to the constitutive negative transmembrane potential present in all cells in their

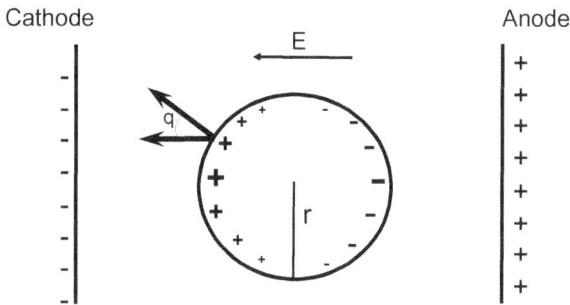

**Figure 7.3.** Ionic charge density inside the cell membrane caused by an external electric field.

basal state. Thus, a more significant polarization and permeabilization is observed on the anode side, where the absolute values of the two constitutive and electro-induced transmembrane potentials add up. This has been confirmed by ultrafast videomicroscopy at the single-cell level.

Noteworthy, the surface charge density of ionic charges which accumulate at the membrane is proportional to the ratio of the total amount of intracellular ions (which is correlated to the cell volume) divided by the cell surface area. Hence, the cell membrane's surface charge density and resulting $\Delta V_m$ depend on the cell dimension or radius $r$. The crucial consequences of this "radius effect" are multiple and provide clues regarding the efficiency of the technology:

(1) Large cells are permeabilized at lower and potentially less toxic electric fields, which explains the exceptional efficiency of electrotransfer on myofibers; also, myotubes are permeabilized at lower fields than their stem cells (the so-called "satellite cells"), which is advantageous for fast tissue repair. Indeed, skeletal muscle cells are electrotransferred using electric fields ranging from 100 to 200 V/cm, while 500–1000 V/cm fields are used for cancer cells, and fields of 5000 V/cm are applied for bacteria.

(2) Small intracellular compartments are not permeabilized. This spares mitochondria, whose functions depend on the internal mitochondrial membrane polarization, and also avoids leakage from lysosomes, which could harm or potentially kill the electrotransferred cells.

(3) Extracellular matrixes are not affected, which also contributes to adequate tissue repair of damages suffered by cells that have undergone excessive permeabilization. The absence of scars and exquisite tissue repair after electrotransfer has been confirmed in various species, including dogs.

It is generally accepted that membrane destabilization and the resulting permeability to hydrophilic external molecules are necessary for DNA electrotransfer to occur. Such permeabilization has been evaluated by measuring the uptake by muscle cells of a small hydrophilic complex of ethylenediaminetetraacetic acid (EDTA) to chromium-51. As shown in Figure 7.4(A), the cell membrane permeabilization to Cr-EDTA remained similar regardless of whether Cr-EDTA was injected 30 s before or after delivery of pulses. In contrast, DNA must strictly be present during the delivery of electric pulses for transfection to occur (Figure 7.4(B)).

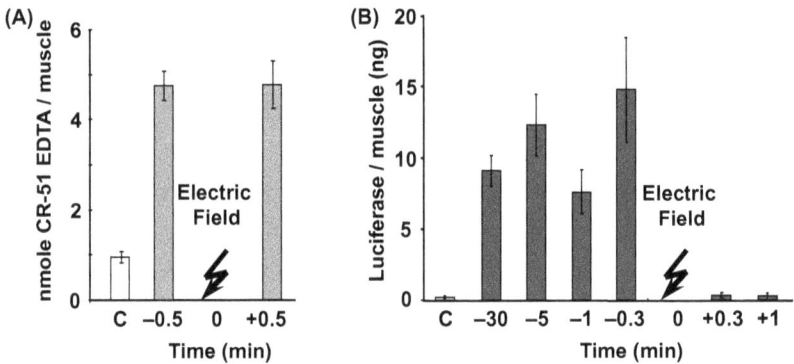

**Figure 7.4.**    Effect of DNA injection time. In (A), the uptake of the Cr-51/EDTA complex is identical whether electropermeabilization is performed shortly before or after the administration of Cr-51/EDTA, which indicates that the permeabilization effect is durable for at least 30 s. In (B), the expression of the luciferase transgene is observed only when plasmid DNA is present during electric field delivery. This means that the electric field must exert a direct effect on DNA (i.e., electrophoresis) for gene transfer to occur. In coherence with that result, the efficacy of electrotransfer is strictly proportional to the duration of the pulse trains, up to a certain level under the toxicity thershold (not shown).

Figure 7.4 demonstrates the direct electrophoretic effect of the electric field on the DNA molecule during the electrotransfer process. Thus, DNA transfer by electric pulses appears to be a two-component phenomenon requiring not only cell "permeabilization" but also the active electrophoresis of DNA during the electric pulse stimulation, which is the result of the effect of the electric field on the negatively charged DNA. This is schematized in Figure 7.5.

The electrophoretic component of DNA electrotransfer has been demonstrated *in vitro* by an experiment in which transfection efficiency on a cell in monolayer was found to vary depending on whether the electric field applied had a polarity-inducing DNA electrophoresis toward the cells or away from the cells. Electrophoresis of DNA has several possible effects, such as promoting the movement of DNA into permeabilized cells and favoring the insertion of DNA in a membrane destabilized by an electric field.

The association of permeabilization and electrophoresis of DNA during electrotransfer has been further highlighted by studying the

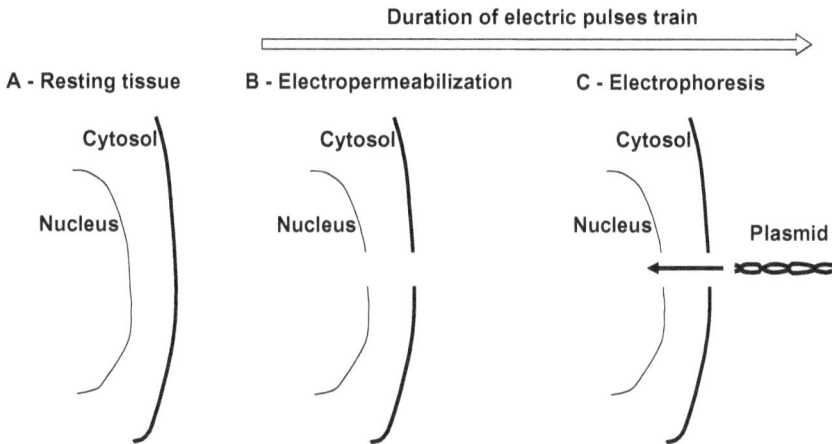

**Figure 7.5.**   (A) Two-component mechanism of DNA electrotransfer mediated by the external electric field: (B) electropermeabilization allows the transmembrane crossing of hydrophilic molecules such as plasmid DNA, and (C) electrophoresis promotesDNA migration toward and within the cell to the nucleus.

combination of a high-voltage permeabilizing pulse of short duration (permeabilizing pulse) with a low-voltage non-permeabilizing electrophoretic pulse of long duration (Figure 7.6). Only the permeabilization pulse followed by the electrophoretic pulse led to highly efficient gene transfer. This indicates that the electrophoretic effect of a low-voltage pulse can contribute to an efficient transfection, provided that the cell membrane has been previously destabilized by a permeabilizing pulse. The importance of cell permeabilization was also studied using magnetic resonance imaging with a contrast agent, gadolinium complex (Gd-DTPA). Results show that the zone of permeabilization for the Gd-DTPA complex is similar to the zone of expression for an electrotransferred plasmid encoding $\beta$-galactosidase.

In addition to the characteristics of the electric pulses, several other factors may be critical for optimizing the efficacy of electrotransfer, thus enabling clinical applications.

Decreasing plasmid size by using minicircles or miniplasmids strongly increases transfection efficiency. These minimal-size plasmids have been presented in Section 5.2 of Chapter 5. The *in vivo* injection into

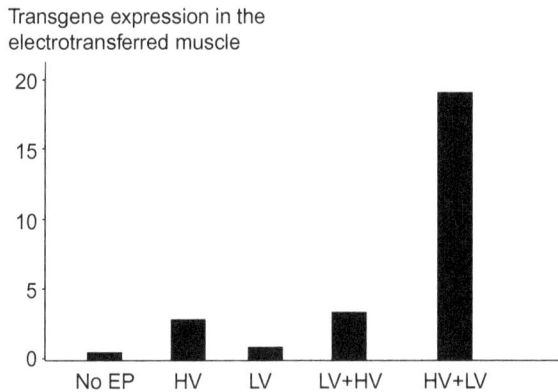

Transgene expression in the
electrotransferred muscle

**Figure 7.6.** The two-component mechanism of DNA electrotransfer is revealed by varying the succession of permeabilizing and electrophoretic pulses. HV: permeabilizing high-voltage pulse of 800 V/cm, 100 $\mu$s. LV: electrophoretic low-voltage pulse of 80 V/cm, 100 ms. No EP: absence of electric pulses. Only HV followed by LV is successful, i.e., permeabilization followed by electrophoresis.

mouse cranial-tibial muscle or into human head and neck carcinoma grafted in nude mice resulted in 13–50 times more reporter gene expression with minicircles than with the classical full size plasmid or larger plasmids. Histological analysis of muscle revealed that there were more transfected myofibers containing minicircles than those with classical full size plasmid. As shown in Figure 7.7, the efficacy of *in vivo* electrotransfer is inversely correlated with the size of the vector.

Electroporation is a physical approach, and as such almost any tissue in a living animal could be targeted to deliver DNA using this method: tumors, bladder, brain, arteries, cornea, heart, joints, liver, lungs, skin, etc. However, the transfection efficiency varies among different tissues. Muscle and skin as tissue targets have shown value in DNA vaccines and gene therapy protocols.

Skeletal muscle constitutes a large, easily accessible volume of tissue in which DNA electroporation is exceptionally efficient. Another interest of skeletal muscle is that muscle fibers are post-mitotic differentiated cells displaying a long lifespan, potentially allowing long-term expression in transfected cells, more than a year in the absence of regeneration due to

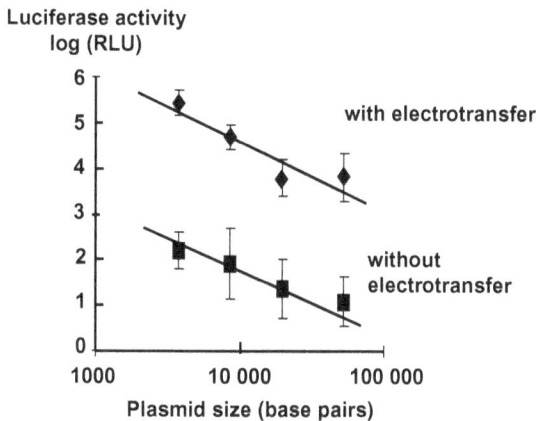

**Figure 7.7.** The level of transfection into tibial cranial skeletal muscle is inversely correlated to plasmid size and is strongly increased by electrotransfer (more than two logs, i.e., 100-fold). The reporter gene used is the firefly luciferase reporter gene, whose activity can be measured by the luminescence reaction in the presence of the substrate luciferin.

injury or cytotoxic immune response. This latter point is of great importance since electroporation does not lead to DNA integration but rather to
episomal localization of the plasmid. Finally, skeletal muscle consists of
thousands of cylindrical muscle fibers bound together by connective
tissue through which run blood vessels and nerves. This constitutes an
abundant blood-vascular system. Skeletal muscle is therefore able to produce secreted proteins with functional post-translational modifications
which can easily reach the bloodstream, including large proteins such as
antibodies.

## 7.2 Clinical Applications of Electrotransfer/ Electrogene Transfer

Treatment of cancer remains a viable target for electroporation-based
therapies. Many studies have evaluated the effectiveness of delivering
plasmids with a variety of effector genes. These include tumor suppres-
sors, immunomodulating agents, inhibitors of cell growth, and pro-
apoptotic agents. Several of these studies have also evaluated combination
approaches (delivery of both drugs and genes).

Immunogenotherapy has been the most investigated approach, including in human clinical trials. It is based on the local transfection of an
immunostimulatory cytokine encoding plasmid, such as IL12. The electric pulse delivery has been shown to induce locally tumor cell death,
leading to the release of tumor antigens and their uptake by professional
antigen-presenting dendritic cells. This specific antitumoral adaptive
immune response is potentiated by immune system activation through the
local production of inflammatory cytokines by transfected surviving cells.
With this strategy, tumor regression has been observed in humans not only
at the electrotransfer site but also on distant tumor nodules. The first clinical trial utilized *in vivo* electrotransfer to deliver interleukin-12 (hIL-12)
gene directly into cutaneous lesions of patients with malignant melanoma.
Other potentially valuable cytokines include IFNα for both melanoma and
squamous cell carcinoma, IL-15 for melanoma, or IL-21 for rectal carcinoma. Combination approaches associating several cytokine genes have

also been tested in clinical trials (B7.1 complementary cDNA with either GMCSF or IL-12 cDNA) to treat fibrosarcoma and squamous cell carcinoma, respectively.

Another anticancer *in vivo* electrotransfer approache, which has been clinically tested, delivers the telomerase cDNA in order to foster an immune response against this protein, which is highly overexpressed in tumor cells. Another anticancer DNA vaccine tested in humans uses the intramuscular electrotransfer of a plasmid encoding a tetanus toxin domain fused to prostate-specific membrane antigen PSMA, which has been delivered to patients with recurrent prostate cancer.

Genetic vaccines, achieved through the electrotransfer of plasmid DNA, are currently being actively developed for the treatment of infectious diseases, such as chronic Human Papillomavirus (HPV) infections. Chronic HPV infection by high-risk HPV serotypes is the main cause of cervical dysplasia in a woman's pelvic cavity. This infection is also associated with cancers of the genitals, and they frequently occur in the oropharynx (mouth and throat) in men. While a prophylactic HPV vaccine is available, it is not systematically delivered to the population. In a gene electrotransfer protocol, it is considered that the increased expression of HPV antigen and the local inflammation associated with electropermeabilization induce a superior immune response, leading to viral regression in the chronically infected tissue. Phase II studies, using either intramuscular or intradermal electrotransfer of HPV-6 and HPV-11 genes, have led to promising results. The FDA has provided feedback that data from the completed INO-3107 Phase 1/2 trial could support a Biological License Application under the Accelerated Approval Program.

The clinical trial concerning *in vivo* gene therapy for hearing disorders through electrotransfer of neurotrophic factor genes to the cochlea is described in Section 5.2 of Chapter 5. Another *in vivo* electrotransfer application is based on the transfection of the eye ciliary muscle. The ciliary muscle is then used as a protein factory to produce therapeutic proteins such as either an anti-inflammatory factor, soluble TNF-α receptor for the treatment of uveitis, or an anti-angiogenic anti-VEGF factor for wet age-related macular degeneration.

Other progressing clinical gene-electrotransfer applications concern *ex vivo* approaches. Electrotransfer is being used together with the Sleeping Beauty transposon technology to generate CAR-T cells in non-viral adoptive immunotherapy protocols (Chapter 8). In a different field, electrotransfer and Sleeping Beauty transposon are being investigated for the treatment of wet age-related macular degeneration (wet AMD). A few thousand cells are collected from the patient's iris or cornea. These cells are transfected by *in vitro* electrotransfer of a miniplasmid encoding the antiangiogenic Pigmented Epithelium Derived Factor (PEDF). After this stable transfection step, the iris or corneal cells are implanted in the vicinity of the patient's macula. In preclinical studies, this approach has demonstrated robust anti-angiogenic efficacy, enabling it to halt the angiogenic progression in the macula of wet-AMD disease models.

## 7.3  Magnetofection

Magnetofection introduces nucleic acids into cells by associating them with magnetic nanoparticles. These molecular complexes are then concentrated and transported into cells, with the support of an applied magnetic field. The magnetic nanoparticles are typically made of iron oxide. They are delivered into the systemic circulation via intravenous injections or administered near the target site in the body, and a strong magnetic field is applied around the target tissue, which facilitates magnetic nanoparticles to accumulate locally.

Advantages of magnetofection include its high efficiency, targeted delivery capacity, and reduced toxicity due to lowered nucleic acid dosage requirements. While magnetic nanoparticles open the possibility to deliver a controlled accumulation and release of these particles and to track these particles by magnetic resonance imaging, magnetofection efficacy depends on further intracellular internalization and endosomal escape of the magnetic nanosystems. Indeed, the magnetic concentration effect increases transfection only when DNA or RNA drugs are complexed with chemical vectors such as cationic lipids, cationic polymers, or LNPs (Chapter 6). Polyethyleneimine (PEI) is the most popular transfection agent so far, which has been associated with magnetic particles.

Magnetofection holds promise for various clinical applications, such as gene replacement therapy, cancer treatment (for instance, by enhancing the delivery of antioncogenic siRNA), vaccines, and regenerative medicine by delivering genes that promote tissue repair and regeneration, including in neurological disorders such as Parkinson's disease. Tissues which have been transfected using this technique in preclinical animal studies include subcutaneous tumors, deep tumors, lungs, hearts, testes, livers, brains, hind legs, and vessels. Magnetic nanoparticles might also be conjugated with targeting moieties, such as transferrin for crossing the blood–brain barrier, or galactose for targeting the liver. The *in vivo* use of magnetic nanoparticles delivered to the blood circulation is, however, hampered by interactions with blood components, such as opsonizing proteins, which might cause rapid blood clearance and elimination by the reticuloendothelial system, especially liver Kupffer cells.

## 7.4 Laser-Based Gene Transfection

The plasma membrane of mammalian cells can be transiently permeabilized by optical means, thus allowing the penetration of exogenous genes. Laser-mediated gene transfection is attractive for targeted gene therapy because of the high spatial controllability of the laser energy. Of value is also the possibility to deliver a laser beam through an optical fiber, thus allowing for highly precise, catheter-based gene transfer into deep tissues. Several laser-based gene transfection techniques have been implemented, including the following: optoinjection, transfection by laser-induced stress waves, photochemical internalization, and selective cell targeting using light-absorbing particles. These techniques are mainly envisioned for *in vitro* gene transfection.

**Optoinjection:** In general, for optoinjection, a single cell is directly irradiated by a focused laser beam, and consequently, this cell alone is loaded with exogenous molecules. Optoinjection uses nanosecond-duration pulses and laser microscope systems, allowing perforation of cells with submicrometer sizes in a single shot of a few nanosecond laser pulses. Another approach uses the blue beam of an argon laser (488 nm) targeted to the cell membrane in the presence of phenol red, a common component of cell culture media, which is used as a non-cytotoxic light-absorbing dye. At the site of the beam impact, the permeability of the cell membrane is modified, which allows plasmid DNA to enter.

**Transfection by laser-induced stress waves:** Short laser pulses generate stress waves, which induce in cultured cells a transient increase in cell plasma membrane permeability. Although this can be detrimental for biomedical applications of pulsed high-powered lasers, the effect can be used to deliver genes to cells. The impulse of the shock wave might change the permeability not only of the cell plasma membrane but also that of the nuclear membrane, thus allowing the transfer of molecules directly into the nucleus. By using the laser-induced stress wave method, a large number of cells can be treated simultaneously. In addition, the treatment of deep-located tissue is possible because a stress wave can be efficiently propagated into tissue. *In vivo,* targeted gene transfer into skin and the central nervous system *using* laser-induced stress waves has been described. However, stress waves induce cell injury, which must be must be considered when implementing this technique.

**Photochemical internalization:** Photosensitizing molecules, such as porphyrins, have been proposed as gene delivery agents. These compounds are widely employed in clinical settings as part of photodynamic therapy protocols for the treatment of cancer, including skin cancers or precancer actinic keratosis. Photochemical-induced internalization is based on light activation of a photosensitizer, which has been previously endocytosed together with the genetic material. Light induces the formation of reactive oxygen species, of which singlet oxygen is the predominant form. Singlet oxygen oxidizes endosome membrane components and induces the release of the genetic material into the cytosol. The potential toxicity of the photosensitizer on the genetic material must however be considered.

**Selective cell targeting with light-absorbing particles:** In this technique, light-absorbing particles are conjugated with cells, which are subsequently irradiated by a laser within a plasmid-containing medium. This leads to selective gene transfer into the targeted cell. Iron-oxide-containing latex microspheres, 20 nm immunogold particles, or 15–30 nm antibody-conjugated gold nanoparticles have been described for selective cell targeting due to their light absorption capacity.

## 7.5  Hydrodynamic Gene Delivery

Hydrodynamic gene delivery is a method based on the application of a high pressure to the vasculature through the rapid injection of a large volume of solution containing a nucleic acid. Plasmid DNA, mRNA, ASO, or siRNA can be delivered *in vivo* to tissue parenchymal cells via the hydrodynamic pressure generated by injection. Hydrodynamic gene delivery represents an efficient, convenient, and easy method for *in vivo* gene transfer in animals, primarily in mice. Most of the uses described concern the high efficiency of plasmid DNA delivery to the mouse liver via tail vein injection; however, proofs of concept for liver hydrodynamic delivery in larger animals, such as pigs or dogs, have also been reported. In addition, delivery to limb skeletal muscle using a tourniquet has been demonstrated in animals.

The efficacy in mouse of plasmid delivery by tail-vein injection results from the following sequence of related events. (1) The bolus injection of a large volume of DNA solution induces cardiac congestion (2) This causes an accumulation of the injected solution in the inferior vena cava resulting in increased intravascular pressure. (3) This accumulation leads to retrograde flow of the DNA solution into the hepatic vein and liver vasculature. (4) This retrograde flow induces hydrodynamic forces which enlarge the liver endothelial sinusoid fenestrae and allow direct access of plasmid DNA to hepatocytes surface. (5) The local pressure induces transient pores in the hepatocyte plasma membrane, thus leading to intracellular plasmid delivery.

Hydrodynamic gene delivery has several advantages, such as high efficiency in the liver: About 40% of hepatocytes are transfected with a single injection of 50 $\mu$g of plasmid DNA in saline through a mouse tail vein over a period of 5 s in a volume equal to 8–10% of the animal's body weight. In addition, the technique allows the delivery of a relatively large volume of DNA solution. However, this technology has limitations because it causes temporary tissue damage due to high pressure and induces cell death due to the transient pores. In addition, by applying the same protocol in terms of volume and speed of injection, various intratissular pressures have been reported, dependent on tissue composition among different individuals. Especially, the fibrotic state might represent a particularly crucial factor in the inter-individual variability for further development of this technique to human clinical use with a balloon catheter delivering the plasmid to specific liver lobes.

The general safety considerations for future clinical use cover transient effects, such as reduced activity, decreased breathing, tissue damage, and recorded increased release of liver enzymes. For further clinical use, it is thus important to standardize a protocol where a similar intravascular pressure is imposed within a controlled volume of tissue in different patients, each having varying tissue composition and fibrotic status.

Loco-regional hydrodynamic delivery can be achieved by the insertion of an injecting device into a defined vasculature. This has been performed by inserting a catheter into a vessel appropriate for the target organ, such as the renal vein for the kidney, the dorsalis pedis vein for muscle tissue, and the superior mesenteric vein for the pancreas. In the liver, delivery to a single lobe has been achieved by using an inflatable balloon in order to block counterflow. Image-guided and region-specific hydrodynamic gene delivery to the liver has been established in pigs, dogs, and baboons by inserting the balloon catheter into the hepatic vein.

In order to obtain a standardized intravascular pressure, a retro-controlled electric injection device has been proposed, which instantaneously monitors the intravascular pressure and adapts the volume injection rate using a pump in order to achieve the desired safe and efficient intravascular pressure and hydrodynamic process (Figure 7.8).

The gene delivery efficiency of the hydrodynamic procedure depends on the capillary structure, the fibrotic state, and the hydrodynamic force applied to the interior of the vasculature. Fenestrated capillaries or

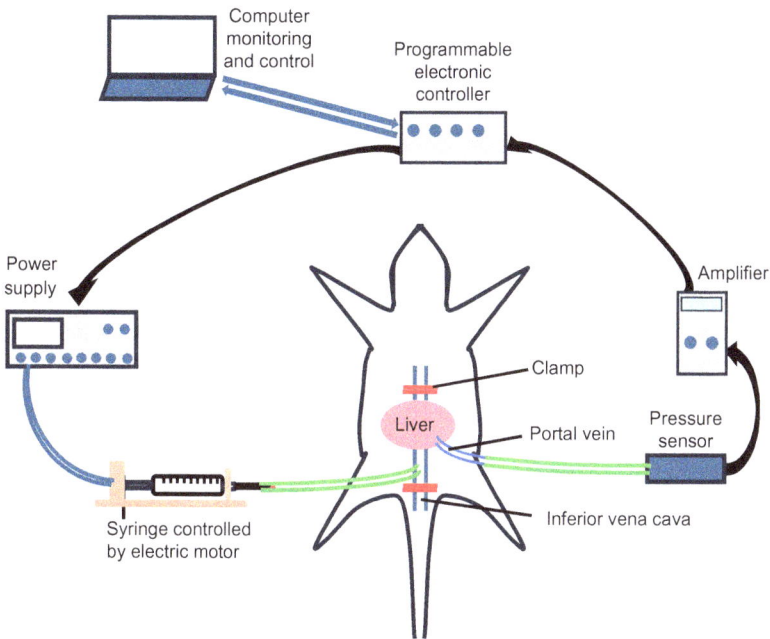

**Figure 7.8.** Retro-controlled hydrodynamic delivery. The rate of plasmid injection by the syringe is determined by the loop system in order to ensure an efficient and safe pressure within the liver. The inferior vena cava is clamped during the procedure.

*Source*: Adapted from Yokoo *et al.* (2016).

sinusoids, which are observed in the liver, are more favorable for hydro-dynamic delivery than continuous capillaries of other tissues, such as muscle tissue. However, the hydrodynamic delivery of naked plasmid DNA into a limb muscle has been well established. One procedure involves placing a tourniquet over the proximal part of the target limb to block all blood flow, followed by the rapid injection of a large volume of plasmid DNA. This promotes plasmid DNA extravasation and its access to the parenchymal muscle cells (myotubes). In this regard, the hydrody-namic limb vein (HLV) injection, also referred to as "limb perfusion", has been proposed as a promising route for either viral or non-viral gene delivery to the skeletal muscle. The HLV approach results in a transient increase in blood pressure and facilitates homogeneous and widespread gene distribution necessary to whole-muscle correction. The HLV method has demonstrated good tolerance in patients with muscular dystrophy.

Finally, other physical techniques based on pressure forces have been proposed, such as needle-free jet injection and particle bombardment gene transfer.

## 7.6  Sonoporation and Acoustothermal Transfection

Ultrasound is an acoustic method widely used in clinical practice for *in vivo* bioimaging. Well-defined, tolerated protocols are available. Many attempts to use ultrasound for mediating drug and gene delivery have been described, with several clinical trial applications for delivering anticancer drugs into tumors. Ultrasounds used in medical echography, cannot on their own effectively disrupt cell plasma membranes *in vivo*. Hence, ultrasound-based delivery techniques use echo-responsive microbubbles, whose resonance induces transient pores in the plasma membranes. A refinement of this technology is the use of high-intensity, focused ultrasound technique (HIFU), another non-invasive and acoustic method which involves the use of a piezoelectric transducer to deliver high-energy pulses in a spatially coordinated manner while minimizing damage to tissue outside the target area.

The mechanism of ultrasound-mediated gene delivery is based on ultrasound-induced radiation force, which induces an increased pressure; as a key effect, it results in acoustic cavitation. Acoustic cavitation describes the process by which pressure field differences in the targeted tissue lead to the formation, oscillation, and collapse of microbubbles. While ultrasound administered at a low intensity causes shear stress on nearby structures, ultrasound administered at high intensity leads to the formation of jet streams and shock waves. In both cases, this leads to the creation of transient reversible pores in cells plasma membrane and an increase in cellular permeability, thereby allowing intracellular delivery of plasmids, DNA, ASOs, or siRNA (Figure 7.9).

This process of pore formation during sonoporation, which allows for increased particle uptake in target tissues and the crossing of intercellular

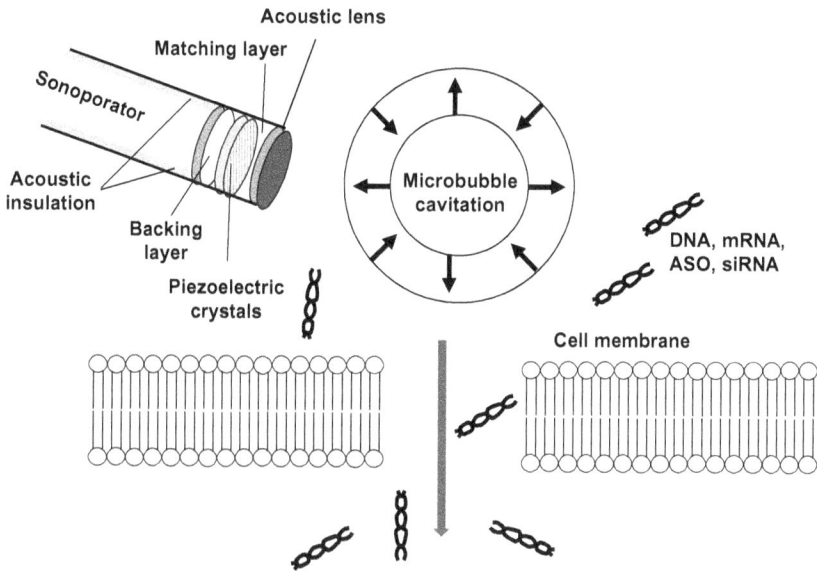

**Figure 7.9.** Schematic diagram depicting sonoporation gene delivery. The sonoporator, or "transducer," induces microbubble acoustic cavitation, which creates a shock wave that destabilizes the cell membrane and allows gene therapy drugs to penetrate through the transient pores.

and intracellular barriers, is greatly enhanced in the presence of gas-filled microbubbles, which are usually used as contrast agents for ultrasound imaging. Under ultrasonic stimulation, oscillating microbubbles contract and expand, and eventually collapse, inducing a negative acoustic pressure. The microbubbles induce the surrounding liquid into motion and create shearing forces. Collapsed microbubbles generate shock waves and micro-jet streams in the fluid.

The deformation and collapse of microbubbles depend on the acoustic energy field delivered, which is related to the ultrasound parameters. For instance, by modulating this parameter, it has been possible to target plasmid delivery either to the hepatocytes using high energy ($110$ W/cm$^2$, $150$ $\mu$s pulse duration) or to liver sinusoid endothelial cells using low energy ($50$ W/cm$^2$, $150$ $\mu$s pulse duration). It was shown that low-energy-mediated plasmid delivery to endothelial cells leads to a higher production of clotting factor VIII, which may be relevant for gene therapy treatment of hemophilia.

Several publications have reported that sonoporation-mediated gene delivery into tumors, such as delivering the inflammatory cytokine gene IL-12, can foster an immune rejection of the tumors.

An interesting recent work has reported a bubble-free acoustothermal transfection technique, which takes advantage of the combined acoustic and thermal effects induced by surface acoustic waves to enhance cell membrane and nuclear envelope transient permeability. This enables safe, efficient, and high-throughput transfection of hard-to-transfect cells. The technique applies acoustic forces on cells to perforate them and takes advantage of the thermal pulses induced by the viscous damping of acoustic waves. This efficient technique is easily scalable, allowing for the transfection of several million cells per minute.

# Bibliography

## *Electrotransfer/Electrogene transfer*

Bigey P, Bureau MF, Scherman D. *In vivo* plasmid DNA electrotransfer. *Curr Opin Biotechnol.* 2002 Oct;13(5):443–7. doi: 10.1016/s0958-1669(02)00377-4.

Bureau MF, Scherman D. Plasmid DNA electrotransfer: a new non viral method for gene therapy in oncology. *Technol Cancer Res Treat.* 2002 Apr;1(2): 149–52. doi: 10.1177/153303460200100208.

Escriou V, Ciolina C, Helbling-Leclerc A, Wils P, Scherman D. Cationic lipid-mediated gene transfer: analysis of cellular uptake and nuclear import of plasmid DNA. *Cell Biol Toxicol.* 1998 Mar;14(2):95–104. doi: 10.1023/a:1007425803756.

Guo S, Donate A, Basu G, Lundberg C, Heller L, Heller R. Electro-gene transfer to skin using a noninvasive multielectrode array. *J Control Release.* 2011 May 10;151(3):256–62. doi: 10.1016/j.jconrel.2011.01.014.

Neumann E, Schaefer-Ridder M, Wang Y, Hofschneider PH. Gene transfer into mouse lyoma cells by electroporation in high electric fields. *EMBO J.* 1982;1(7):841–5. doi: 10.1002/j.1460-2075.1982.tb01257.x.

Rochard A, Scherman D, Bigey P. Genetic immunization with plasmid DNA mediated by electrotransfer. *Hum Gene Ther*. 2011 Jul;22(7):789–98. doi: 10.1089/hum.2011.092.

## *Clinical applications of electrotransfer/electrogene transfer*

Bloquel C, Bejjani R, Bigey P, *et al*. Plasmid electrotransfer of eye ciliary muscle: principles and therapeutic efficacy using hTNF-alpha soluble receptor in uveitis. *FASEB J*. 2006 Feb;20(2):389–91. doi: 10.1096/fj.05-4737fje.

Johnen S, Harmening N, Marie C, Scherman D, Izsvák Z, Ivics Z, Walter P, Thumann G. Electroporation-based genetic modification of primary human pigment epithelial cells using the Sleeping Beauty transposon system. *J Vis Exp*. 2021 Feb 4;(168). doi: 10.3791/61987.

Kropp M, Harmening N, Bascuas T, *et al*. GMP-grade manufacturing and quality control of a non-virally engineered advanced therapy medicinal product for personalized treatment of age-related macular degeneration. *Biomedicines*. 2022 Nov 1;10(11):2777. doi: 10.3390/biomedicines10112777.

Pinyon JL, von Jonquieres G, Crawford EN, *et al*. Neurotrophin gene augmentation by electrotransfer to improve cochlear implant hearing outcomes. *Hear Res*. 2019 Sep 1;380:137–149. doi: 10.1016/j.heares.2019.06.002.

Trollet C, Bloquel C, Scherman D, Bigey P. Electrotransfer into skeletal muscle for protein expression. *Curr Gene Ther*. 2006 Oct;6(5):561–78. doi: 10.2174/156652306778520656.

Trollet C, Scherman D, Bigey P. Delivery of DNA into muscle for treating systemic diseases: advantages and challenges. *Methods Mol Biol*. 2008;423:199–214. doi: 10.1007/978-1-59745-194-9_14.

## *Magnetofection*

Azadpour B, Aharipour N, Paryab A, Omid H, Abdollahi S, Madaah Hosseini H, Malek Khachatourian A, Toprak MS, Seifalian AM. Magnetically assisted viral transduction (magnetofection) medical applications: an update. *Biomater Adv*. 2023 Nov;154:213657. doi: 10.1016/j.bioadv.2023.213657.

Sizikov AA, Nikitin PI, Nikitin MP. Magnetofection *in vivo* by nanomagnetic carriers systemically administered into the bloodstream. *Pharmaceutics*. 2021 Nov 14;13(11):1927. doi: 10.3390/pharmaceutics13111927.

## Laser-based gene transfection

Ogura M, Sato S, Nakanishi K, Uenoyama M, Kiyozumi T, Saitoh D, Ikeda T, Ashida H, Obara M. *In vivo* targeted gene transfer in skin by the use of laser-induced stress waves. *Lasers Surg Med.* 2004;34(3):242–8. doi: 10.1002/lsm.20024.

Yao C, Zhang ZX, Rahmanzadeh R, Hüttmann G. Laser-based gene transfection and gene therapy. *IEEE Trans Nanobioscience.* 2008 Jul;7(2):111–9. doi: 10.1109/TNB.2008.2000742.

## Hydrodynamic gene delivery

Fan Z, Kocis K, Valley R, Howard JF Jr, *et al.* High-pressure transvenous perfusion of the upper extremity in human muscular dystrophy: a safety study with 0.9% saline. *Hum Gene Ther.* 2015 Sep;26(9):614–21. doi: 10.1089/hum.2015.023.

Hagstrom JE, Hegge J, Zhang G, Noble M, Budker V, Lewis DL, Herweijer H, Wolff JA. A facile nonviral method for delivering genes and siRNAs to skeletal muscle of mammalian limbs. *Mol Ther.* 2004 Aug;10(2):386–98. doi: 10.1016/j.ymthe.2004.05.004.

Le Guen YT, Le Gall T, Midoux P, Guégan P, Braun S, Montier T. Gene transfer to skeletal muscle using hydrodynamic limb vein injection: current applications, hurdles and possible optimizations. *J Gene Med.* 2020 Feb;22(2):e3150. doi: 10.1002/jgm.3150.

Liu F, Song Y, Liu D. Hydrodynamics-based transfection in animals by systemic administration of plasmid DNA. *Gene Ther.* 1999 Jul;6(7):1258–66. doi: 10.1038/sj.gt.3300947.

Pastor M, Quiviger M, Pailloux J, Scherman D, Marie C. Reduced heterochromatin formation on the pFAR4 miniplasmid allows sustained transgene expression in the mouse liver. *Mol Ther Nucleic Acids.* 2020 Sep 4;21:28–36. doi: 10.1016/j.omtn.2020.05.014.

Quiviger M, Arfi A, Mansard D, Delacotte L, Pastor M, Scherman D, Marie C. High and prolonged sulfamidase secretion by the liver of MPS-IIIA mice following hydrodynamic tail vein delivery of antibiotic-free pFAR4 plasmid vector. *Gene Ther.* 2014 Dec;21(12):1001–7. doi: 10.1038/gt.2014.75.

Suda T, Yokoo T, Kanefuji T, Kamimura K, Zhang G, Liu D. Hydrodynamic delivery: characteristics, applications, and technological advances. *Pharmaceutics.* 2023 Mar 31;15(4):1111. doi: 10.3390/pharmaceutics15041111.

Yokoo T, Kamimura K, Abe H, *et al.* Liver-targeted hydrodynamic gene therapy: recent advances in the technique. *World J Gastroenterol.* 2016 Oct 28;22(40):8862–8. doi: 10.3748/wjg.v22.i40.8862.

## Sonoporation and acoustothermal transfection

Bachu VS, Kedda J, Suk I, Green JJ, Tyler B. High-intensity focused ultrasound: a review of mechanisms and clinical applications. *Ann Biomed Eng.* 2021 Sep;49(9):1975–91. doi: 10.1007/s10439-021-02833-9.

Krut Z, Gazit D, Gazit Z, Pelled G. Applications of ultrasound-mediated gene delivery in regenerative medicine. *Bioengineering (Basel).* 2022 Apr 27;9(5):190. doi: 10.3390/bioengineering9050190.

Lawton SM, Manson MA, Fan MN, Chao TY, Chen CY, Kim P, Campbell C, Cai X, Vander Kooi A, Miao CH. Ultrasound-mediated gene delivery specifically targets liver sinusoidal endothelial cells for sustained FVIII expression in hemophilia A mice. *Mol Ther.* 2024 Apr 3;32(4):969–81. doi: 10.1016/j.ymthe.2024.02.010.

Li Y, Chen Z, Ge S. Sonoporation: underlying mechanisms and applications in cellular regulation. *BIOI.* 2021;2(1):29–36. doi: 10.15212/bioi-2020-0028.

Liu X, Rong N, Tian Z, Rich J, Niu L, Li P, Huang L, Dong Y, *et al.* Acoustothermal transfection for cell therapy. *Sci Adv.* 2024 Apr 19;10(16):eadk1855. doi: 10.1126/sciadv.adk1855.

Mignet N, Marie C, Delalande A, Manta S, Bureau MF, Renault G, Scherman D, Pichon C. Microbubbles for nucleic acid delivery in liver using mild sonoporation. *Methods Mol Biol.* 2019;1943:377–87. doi: 10.1007/978-1-4939-9092-4_25.

Ricci M, Barbi E, Dimitri M, Duranti C, Arcangeli A, Corvi A. Sonoporation, a novel frontier for cancer treatment: a review of the literature. *Appl Sci.* 2024;14(2):515. doi: 10.3390/app14020515.

Sun RR, Noble ML, Sun SS, Song S, Miao CH. Development of therapeutic microbubbles for enhancing ultrasound-mediated gene delivery. *J Control Release.* 2014 May 28;182:111–20. doi: 10.1016/j.jconrel.2014.03.002.

# Chapter 8

# CAR-T Cell Adoptive Immunotherapy

## 8.1 Introduction

Cancer immunotherapy is based on treating tumors indirectly; its aim is not to directly target tumor cells, but rather to use or educate the immune system in order to enable it to eliminate tumor cells through a selectively activated immune reaction.

The spectacular potential of cancer immunotherapy was first illustrated by the extended clinical practice of "checkpoint inhibitors," which are monoclonal antibodies that target specific T-cell activation pathways. Adoptive immunotherapy, which combines cell and gene therapy tools, represents the next breakthrough and most recent transformative strategy to treat incurable cancers.

An overview of the immunological synapse is necessary for understanding checkpoint inhibitors and adoptive immunotherapy. This presentation will be restricted to T lymphocytes (CD4 and CD8) because these are actually the main cells in use for adoptive immunotherapy, whereas other components of the immune response, such as natural killer NK cells or M cells, are already considered for future developments of adoptive immunotherapy.

## 8.2 The Immunological Synapse

When exposed to infected or dysfunctional somatic cells, cytotoxic T cells (CD8+) release the cytotoxins perforin, granzymes, and granulysin. Through the action of perforin, granzymes enter the cytoplasm of the target cell, and their serine protease function triggers the caspase cascade, which involves a series of cysteine proteases that lead to apoptosis (programmed cell death). This process occurs through the formation of the immunological synapse (or immune synapse), which represents the interacting contact zone between a T lymphocyte and an antigen-presenting cell (APC, also called dendritic cell) or between a T lymphocyte and a target cell, such as a tumor cell.

At an early initial step, the interaction of several surface proteins of effector T lymphocytes (T4 lymphocytes) with an antigen-presenting cell elicits an activation state which leads to the proliferation and activation of either CD4+ helper T cells or killer CD8+ cytotoxic T cells.

An illustration of an immunological synapse between an APC and a T cell is displayed in Figure 8.1. The major histocompatibility (MHC) complex protein at the surface of an antigen-presenting cell or tumor cell presents a peptide fragment (8–10 amino acid residues for MHC class I and 13–25 residues for MHC class II) derived from a foreign viral protein or tumor cell mutated protein. The T-cell receptor (TCR) binds to the peptide/MHC complex, with each TCR subtype bearing specific recognition capacity for a given peptide/MHC complex. This interaction occurs between an APC or tumor cell and a "naïve" CD4+ T lymphocyte, which will then specialize either into a CD4+ helper T cell if the MHC complex is of class II (i.e., presenting extracellular antigens) or into a cytotoxic CD8+ T cell if the interaction occurs through an MHC class I surface protein. Both CD4 and CD8 molecules at the T-cell surface stabilize the immunological synapse interaction and participate in the phosphorylation of TCR CD3ζ and of zap70 which transduce the activation signal (see the following).

These T lymphocytes will only be activated if the first signal (peptide recognition) is accompanied by the so-called co-stimulatory signals

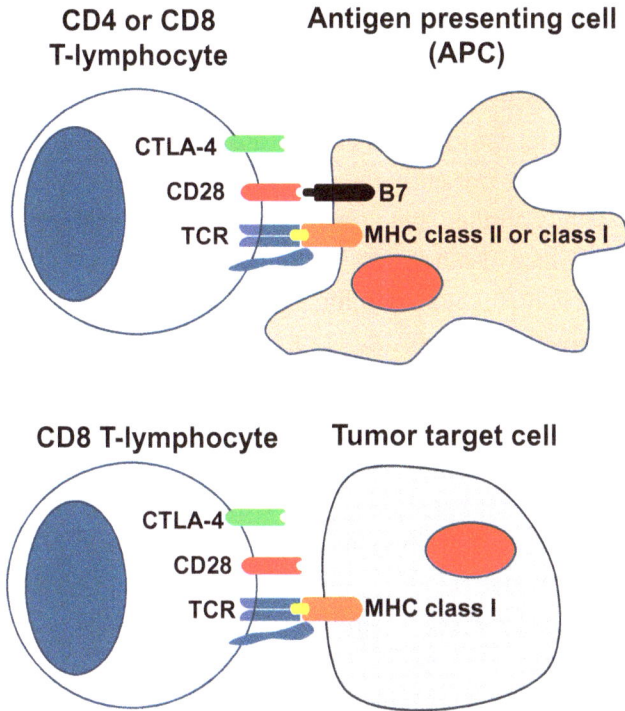

**Figure 8.1.** Key molecular interactions involved in T-cell recognition and activation. Complete activation of effector T cells (either CD4+ or CD8+) requires two signals transmitted by antigen-presenting cells (APC cells). In the first step, a specific peptide antigen (yellow), presented by the major histocompatibility complex (MHC) protein binds to the T-cell receptor (TCR) complex (first signal). The second necessary signal is called "costimulatory signal." One of the main costimulatory pathways (second signal) occurs through the binding of the B7 molecule (black) present on the APC surface to the CD28 receptor expressed on T cells (red). The B7 molecule is also called CD80 for the subtype B7-1 and CD86 for the subtype B7-2. The association of these two signals induces T-lymphocyte proliferation and activates them into the cytotoxic state. Activated cytotoxic T lymphocytes then bind and kill tumor target cells which present the antigen (yellow) through the MHC class I membrane protein. Tumor cells generally do not express the B7-1 costimulatory protein (CD80).

transmitted by B7 molecules. The second signal is delivered to the T lymphocyte by the interaction of accessory T-lymphocyte receptors with ligands on the surface of APC cells. The B7 molecules play this role by binding to CD28 receptors. In the absence of this signal, the lymphocyte becomes tolerant to the antigen. Various adhesion molecules stabilize these interactions. The level of expression of co-stimulatory molecules correlates with the state of maturation of dendritic cells.

Only the co-receptors CD28 and B7 are presented in Figures 8.1 and 8.2 because they are presently the most relevant to the CAR-T cell technology described further, but other very important pathways, such as PD-1 (programmed death) and PD-1 ligand, have been characterized, leading to extensively used mAb for anticancer treatment.

T-cell activation and proliferation is mediated by antigen-specific signals from the TCR–CD4 or TCR–CD8 complex in combination with additional costimulatory signals provided by several co-receptors, such as the extracellular protein CD28, the inducible co-stimulator ICOS, the *cytotoxic T-lymphocyte antigen-4 (CTLA-4)*, the *Programmed Death* receptor (PD-1), and other membrane proteins. While CD28 and ICOS provide positive signals that promote and sustain cytotoxic T-cell responses, CTLA-4 and PD-1 limit the response and antagonize cytotoxic

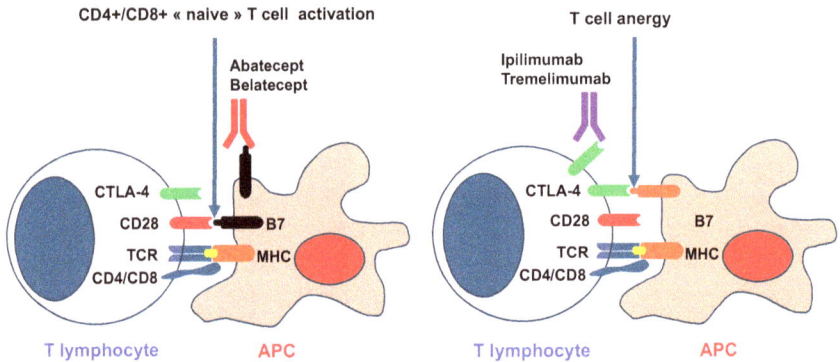

**Figure 8.2.** Molecular interactions involved in T-cell activation or T-cell anergy. When APC-B7 interacts with T-cell CD28, this induces T-cell activation. The monoclonal antibodies Abatecept and Belatecept bind to B7 and prevent this activation. They are clinically used to treat a variety of autoimmune diseases. In contrast, the binding of APC-B7 to T-cell CTLA-4 induces T-cell anergy. This anergizing process is blocked by the monoclonal antibodies Ipilimumab and Tremelimumab, which are called "checkpoint inhibitors." They strongly potentialize T-cell activation and have been proven to be particularly effective association with other anticancer drugs for the treatment of various cancers.

T-cell activation. More precisely, the primary main ligand-receptor pairs are as follows:

- CD28 and B7-1/B7-2 (CD80/CD86): CD28 on T cells binds to B7-1 (CD80) and B7-2 (CD86) on APCs, providing essential signals for T-cell activation and survival.
- ICOS on T cells binds to ICOS-L on APCs, enhancing T-cell proliferation and cytokine production.
- CTLA-4, also on T cells, binds to the same ligands as CD28 but delivers inhibitory signals to downregulate T-cell responses. CTLA-4 stands for "cytotoxic T-lymphocyte-associated protein 4," and it is also designated as CD152, which reflects its identification as part of the cluster of differentiation markers.
- PD-1 on T cells interacts with PD-L1 and PD-L2 on APCs and other cells, leading to the inhibition of T-cell activity and promoting immune tolerance.

These interactions are critical for regulating immune responses, ensuring that T cells are properly activated when necessary and inhibited to prevent overactivation and autoimmunity.

As mentioned, the interaction of APC surface protein B7 with the T-cell costimulatory CD28 is critical for T-cell activation and signal transduction. Remarkably, B7 can interact either with CD28, thus delivering a positive activating signal, or with CTLA-4, which has, in contrast, an inhibitory and anergizing effect in T cells (Figure 8.2). This duality of B7 recognition is essential for the immune system to be controlled and the activation to be terminated: It is the balance between stimulatory and inhibitory co-signals which determines the ultimate nature of T-cell responses, thus controlling inflammation and autoimmunity.

Figure 8.2 allows us to understand the therapeutic rationale for using monoclonal antibodies capable of interfering with the immunological synapse function. The monoclonal antibodies (mAb) Ipilimimab and Tremelimumab target CTLA-4 and inhibit B7 binding to CTLA-4 through a steric effect. Hence, they potentialize T-cell activation and have been shown to be very efficient in association with other anticancer drugs for the treatment of various cancers, such as melanoma, non-small cell lung cancer (NSCLC), renal cell carcinoma, Hodgkin lymphoma, and head-and-neck squamous cell carcinoma. On the other hand, Abatacept and Belatacept mAbs bind to B7 and thus anergize T cells, i.e., they block their activation. They have demonstrated potency in autoimmune disorders, such as various forms of arthritis, including rheumatoid arthritis, and graft rejection. Abatacept is primarily used to treat moderate to severe rheumatoid arthritis in patients who have not responded adequately to other treatments, and also to treat juvenile idiopathic arthritis and graft-versus-host disease (GVHD). Belatacept is used as an immunosuppressive agent in renal transplantation to prevent organ rejection.

## 8.3 T-Cell Receptor Structure and Activation Mechanism

The "TCR complex" schematized in Figure 8.3 comprises eight polypeptides:

(a) The TCR receptor, per se, is a heterodimer composed of the two chains TCRα and TCRβ, which bind to the MHC-borne peptide epitope presented by APCs.

(b) The cluster of differentiation three co-receptor (CD3) helps to activate T cells and consists of four distinct chains: CD3γ, CD3δ, and two CD3ε chains.

(c) Two ζ-chains (zeta-chain) (also called CD3ζ by many authors) are responsible for intracellular signal transduction.

The TCR, CD3γ, CD3δ, and the two CD3ε chains have a very short cytoplasmic tail. On the contrary, the CD3ζ chains possess a much larger cytoplasmic moiety, which contains characteristic sequence motifs for tyrosine phosphorylation called Immunoreceptor Tyrosine-based Activation Motifs (ITAMs). Upon TCR interaction with a peptide/MHC molecule, the ITAMs are phosphorylated, which leads to the binding of zap70 and the initiation of an intracellular signaling pathway. This pathway will not be detailed here; it ultimately leads to IL-2 cytokine

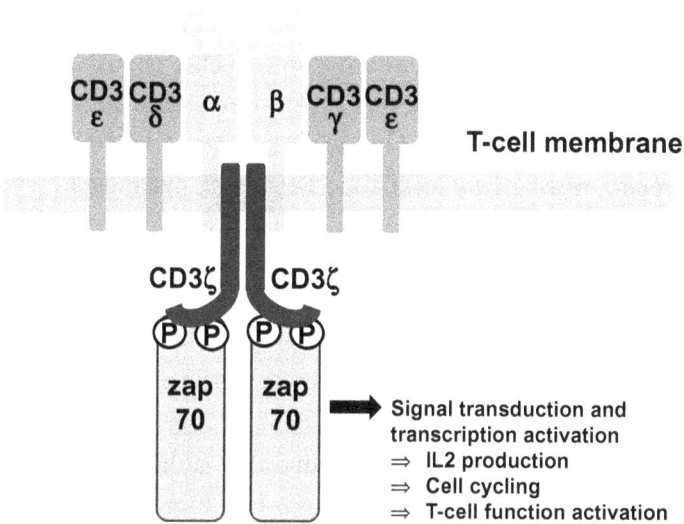

**Figure 8.3.** Molecular assembly of the TCR complex and intracellular signal transduction. The two CD3ζ chains possess long intracellular domains bearing phosphorylation sites called ITAMs. When the TCRα/β binds to the MHC-presented epitope, the ITAMs of the two CD3ζ are phosphorylated, which leads to zap70 binding and intracellular signal transduction. All subsequent intracellular signaling events linked to the TCR complex are mediated through this CD3ζ activation.

production and T-cell function activation. Supplementary stimulatory signals originating from costimulatory molecules, such as CD28, are necessary for the complete activation of the immune response, which involves not only T-cell functional activation but also proliferation and survival enhancement.

## 8.4 General Principle of Adoptive Immunotherapy

In adoptive immunotherapy, tumor cells which express specific antigens are targeted and killed by a selected lymphocyte population. The difficulty arises from the selection of such a competent T-cell population, and this has promoted the development of several revolutionary technologies.

Primary attempts dating from the 1980s consisted of collecting patient tumor tissue, followed by isolating and amplifying from this tissue the

T-cells that were naturally present and involved in the anti-tumor immune response, without any genetic modification. Such a population of amplified tumor-infiltrating lymphocytes (TILs) has shown promising therapeutic results in treating metastatic melanomas and several carcinomas, such as renal, ovarian, colorectal, and pancreatic carcinomas. The problem is that efficient TILs are not found in all tumors and for the same tumor in different patients, and this is the cause of significant interindividual variability in the number and potency of the produced helper and cytotoxic T cells.

The transplantation of non-autologous T cells has also been attempted in hematological malignancies, and allogeneic donor T cells have been shown, in some cases, to eradicate the disease via the graft-versus-leukemia (GVL) effect. But this approach has a low success rate and bears an important risk of graft-versus-host disease (GVHD), in which the grafted lymphocytes destroy cells of the patient, considered as non-self by the graft.

In order to increase the population of tumor-competent T cells, the gene of a TCR bearing a specific affinity for an antigen expressed by tumor cells has been introduced into the patient's own T lymphocytes. This autologous, engineered T-cell population is restricted to a single TCR and is thus potentially of higher efficacy and more widely used than TILs. This strategy was described as being active in myeloma and metastatic melanoma; however, despite its continued pursuit, it suffers from several drawbacks.

First, TCR $\alpha/\beta$ displays a generally low affinity for MHC molecules, and current efforts aim at isolating TCRs with optimal specificity and affinity. Second, since TCR-engineered T lymphocytes require binding to an MHC protein on targeted tumor cells to implement their cytotoxic function, this introduces a limitation linked to human leukocyte antigen (HLA) restriction. The introduced TCR must match the MHC HLA specificity of the patient, which imposes the requirement of identifying multiple TCRs for any given antigen in order to adapt to the specific HLA haplotypes of the patients. Third, tumor cell subpopulations usually evade destruction by down-regulating the expression of MHC molecules on their surfaces. T cells bearring a "chimeric antigen receptor" (CAR-T cells) were introduced to circumvent these shortcomings.

## 8.5 CAR-T Cells Adoptive Immunotherapy

Chimeric antigen receptors (CARs) are fusion proteins engineered to be expressed by a genetically modified T cell. They bind to an antigen, generally a protein, at the surface of a tumor cell, and initiate T-cell activation, thus mimicking a T-cell receptor. The seminal pioneering work was that of Zelig Eshhar at the Weizmann Institute (Israel), who initially called these chimeric antigen receptors "T-bodies." These first-generation CARs showed very promising efficiency in eradicating hematological tumors in animal models, but subsequent clinical trials were disappointing.

A first-generation T body (CAR-T cell) is displayed in Figure 8.4. It results from the fusion of several components, each having a specific

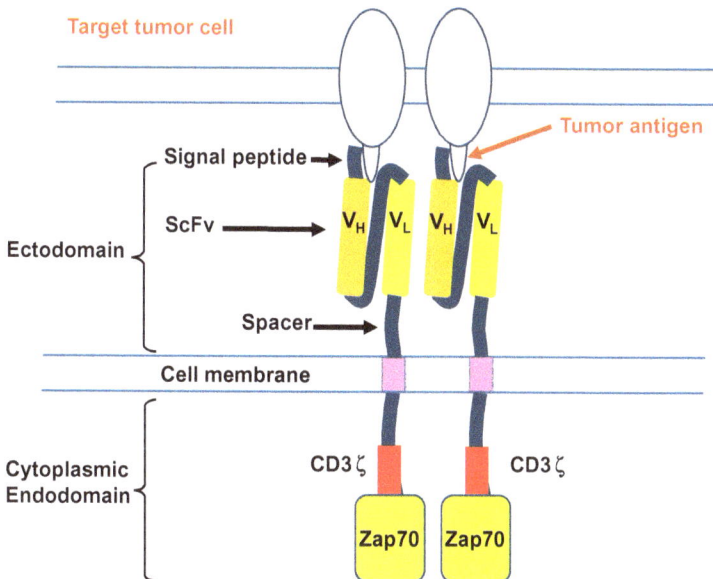

**Figure 8.4.** First-generation chimeric antigen receptor or T-body. The cytoplasmic endodomain derived from the TCR CD3ζ moiety recruits zap70 and initiates T-cell activation/proliferation.

functionality, which makes it possible to optimize an infinite number of combinations for each targeted cell type:

- A signal peptide is necessary to direct the nascent protein to the endoplasmic reticulum and Golgi apparatus lumens and then to the cell surface.
- The ectodomain contains mainly a single-chain variable fragment (ScFv) derived from an antibody, which displays high nanomolar or subnanomolar affinity for the targeted antigen. This ScFv is the key recognition moiety of the epitope/MHC complex. Other ligands to the targeted cell surface proteins can be used.
- A flexible SPACER allows the ScFv or other ligand to orient in different directions, thereby favoring antigen binding. The SPACER is an empirically defined part of the engineered recombinant receptor; however, it plays a key role in the binding efficacy to the targetd antigen. Several often-used fragments consist of the hinge region from IgG1 or portions of CD3.
- The transmembrane domain is a hydrophobic alpha helix usually derived from the original molecule of the signaling endodomain, such as CD3ζ. Alternatively, the transmembrane domain of CD28 or that of the TNFα family has been used.
- The intracellular signaling endodomain protrudes into the cell and transmits the desired activation signal. It was initially speculated that the CD3ζ domain bearing the ITAMs and responsible for initiating intracellular signal transduction would be sufficient to trigger T-cell activation upon binding to a target cell through ScFv recognition. It is assumed that the interaction between two CAR-T receptors associated with two targeted antigens leads to pseudo-dimerization, thereby recruiting two adjacent zap70 molecules and, thus, mimicking in a perfect manner the TCR.

In spite of early promising results in preclinical models, disappointing clinical trials have led to the conclusion that signaling through such first-generation CAR receptors was insufficient to trigger a sufficiently potent and robust immune response. This suggested that it was necessary to mobilize more molecular components of the immunological synapse. Significant advances by several teams, particularly those by C June and M Sadelain, led to the "second-generation" CAR-T cells, which showed extraordinary success in B-lymphocyte malignancies such as acute or chronic lymphocytic leukemia.

The breakthrough came from the addition of another activating moiety to the intracellular fusion endodomain. Typical second- and third-generation chimeric antigen receptors are schematized in Figure 8.5.

The "second-generation" CAR genes add intracellular signaling domains from various costimulatory protein receptors (e.g., CD28, 4-1BB,

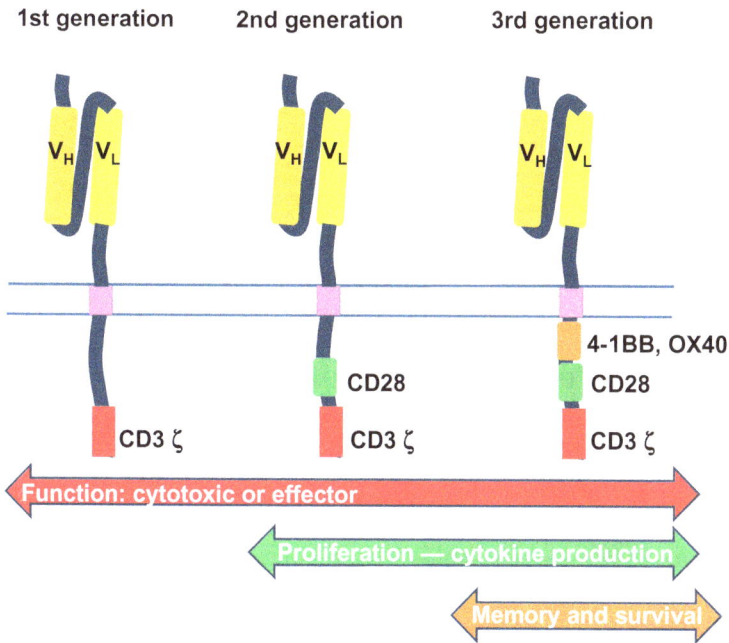

**Figure 8.5.** Successive generations of chimeric antigen receptors. The cytoplasmic endodomain derived from the TCR CD3ζ moiety recruits zap70 and initiates the T-cell activation process. Additional activation is conferred by the intracellular moiety of the CD28 costimulatory molecule, which recruits phosphatidyl inositol 3 (PI3) kinase. Even more potent CAR-T cells can be produced by fusing an additional costimulatory signal in the endodomain, such as 4-1BB, which recruits TRAF2.

and ICOS), leading to more robust antitumor activity, both at preclinical and human clinical levels. The functional properties of CAR-T cells may depend on the co-stimulation signal used. For instance, CD28 promotes T-cell strong and fast proliferation, but with limited persistence, whereas the 4-1 BB costimulatory fusion fragment induces a milder yet more persistent CAR-T cell response.

More recently introduced, the "third-generation" CARs combine multiple signaling domains, such as CD3$\zeta$/CD28/4-1BB or CD3$\zeta$/CD28/OX40, to further increase potency. Importantly, while CD3$\zeta$ recruits zap70 for intracellular signal transduction, the other added costimulatory factors recruit different intracellular relays, such as phosphatidyl inositol 3 kinase (PI3 kinase) for CD28 intracellular fragment and TRAF2 for the 4-1BB intracellular fragment. This results in additive or synergistic activation, and it is generally considered that first-generation CAR receptors induce the differentiated T-cell functions, such as cytotoxicity for CD8 T cells, while second-generation CAR-T cells possess stronger proliferation capacity, mainly due to IL2 production, and third-generation CAR-T cells possess survival and memory capacities. As already mentioned, the "burst effect," or persistent CAR-T cell response, might be modulated by selecting different costimulatory moieties.

## 8.6 CAR-T Cell Production and Administration

The success of the CAR-T cell strategy was built upon many years of meticulously acquired knowledge on T-cell biology and T-cell *in vitro* manipulations. A large number of steps had to be optimized one by one, comprising leukapheresis, apheresis washing, magnetic bead labeling, T-cell enrichment, cell growth formulation, cell stimulation, viral transduction, cell expansion, cell harvest, and quality control testing.

Briefly, blood cells are harvested by leukapheresis from GMCSF-stimulated patients. The preparation is then enriched in T cells. Purity is a critical factor, particularly in ensuring the elimination of any contamination by tumor cells. Various techniques have been used, initially through density gradient separation, followed by centrifugation-based techniques for separation according to cell size. More recent, sophisticated techniques are still based on centrifugation, such as counterflow centrifugal elutriation.

The enriched T cells are then transduced, after a couple of days in culture, in the presence of IL2 and OKT3 antibody (anti-human CD3 murine monoclonal antibody). Stable chromosomal integration of the transgene is an absolute requirement here, since only a few transduced CAR-T cells must undergo a large number of cell division/proliferation, both *in vitro* before IV administration and *in vivo* in order to eliminate patient tumor cells. Thus, most CAR-T cell production processes use a retroviral vector derived from the murine mammary tumor Moloney oncoretrovirus or a HIV-derived lentiviral vector, which promotes random chromosomal integration of the CAR gene. In order to circumvent the risk of insertional oncogenesis, integration must be limited to one or two CAR transgenes per cell, and safer self-inactivated retro/lentiviral vectors are used (Chapter 4).

A less frequently used alternative to lentiviral vectors consists of transfecting a transposon plasmid carrying the CAR sequence associated with a plasmid or mRNA encoding a transposase, such as the "Sleeping Beauty" transposase. The transposase mediates CAR gene stable integration into the T-cell genome in a manner similar to that of a lentivirus, which ensures the stability of expression during the multiple divisions of the *in vitro* and *in vivo* CAR-T cell expansion (Chapter 5).

CAR-T cells are then cultured and expanded *in vitro* for several days (in the presence of IL-2 cytokine using stimulation by anti-CD3/CD28 antibodies coated on beads), and finally injected into the patient along with IL2. Several variants of these techniques have been proposed, and automated devices integrate all these preparation steps within a 7–9 day.

## 8.7 Clinical Results and Applications

A major advantage of CAR-T cells is that they circumvent HLA restriction since no MHC molecule is involved in recognizing the target cell, which results from a direct interaction between the CAR-ScFv moiety and the targeted antigen. In addition, a higher binding affinity is observed with properly selected ScFv when compared to MHC binding. This, and other factors, explain the strikingly efficient results that have been obtained in the first clinical trials concerning acute and chronic lymphoblastic leukemia (ALL and CLL). In these diseases, the bone marrow produces too many B-lymphocytes. Highly robust results have also been obtained in lymphoma, also a blood cancer developed from B-lymphocytes and characterized by enlarged lymph nodes, and in multiple myeloma, a type of cancer that affects plasma cells, which are a type of white blood cell found in the bone marrow. These plasma cells are responsible for producing antibodies that help fight infections. In multiple myeloma, abnormal plasma cells multiply uncontrollably, leading to various health issues.

The CAR targeted marker on B lymphocytes is CD19, which is appealing since it is carried only by B-lymphocytes, whose temporary elimination is not a life-threatening risk. Moreover, the elimination of temporary B cells might allow to avoid an antibody-mediated response against CAR-T cells, which carry a non-self CAR gene. Following preclinical work by Michel Sadelain and colleagues, in 2013, Carl June's group published the results of a clinical trial using CD19 CAR-T cells for acute lymphoblastic leukemia in two patients. Complete remission was observed for the two patients, and in the subsequent two years, five clinical studies reported a range of 70–100% complete remissions in ALL patients with no alternative therapeutic options.

These results generated tremendous excitement, particularly because B-ALL is the most common malignancy in children and because a complete and prolonged remission was observed in patients devoid of any alternative therapeutic options. This was the start of one of the fastest drug development processes in history, and in 2018, two drugs based on anti-CD19 CARs were approved by the FDA for lymphoblastic leukemia and refractory aggressive non-Hodgkin lymphoma. First *tisagenlecleucel* (Kymriah) for the treatment of adult patients with relapsed or refractory (r/r) large B-cell lymphoma after two or more lines of systemic therapy. The indications include diffuse large B-cell lymphoma (DLBCL) not otherwise specified, high-grade B-cell lymphoma, and DLBCL arising from follicular lymphoma. Second, *axicabtagene ciloleucel* (Yescarta) has been the firs CAR-T therapy approved by the FDA for the treatment of adult patients with relapsed or refractory large B-cell lymphoma after two or more lines of systemic therapy.

The CD19 antigen is a protein found on the surface of B cells, which are responsible for recognizing antigens and initiating the immune response. The lymphocyte B-cells can differentiate into plasma cells or memory B cells; B cells are produced by hematopoietic stem cells in the bone marrow, and there are several types of B cells, including naïve B cells, memory B cells, and plasmablasts. When B cells encounter an antigen, they can differentiate into plasma cells or memory B cells.

Up to 2024, CD19-targeted CAR-T cells have been approved for treating relapsed/refractory ALL and large B-cell lymphoma (LBCL), follicular lymphoma (FL), and multiple cell lymphoma (MCL). The approved CD19 CAR-T cell products *tisagenlecleucel* (Kymriah), *lisocabtagene maraleucel* (Breyanzi), and *relmacabtagene autoleucel* (JWCAR029) use the 4-1BB co-stimulatory domain, while the approved products *axicabtagene ciloleucel* (Yescarta)) and *brexucabtagene autoleucel* (Tecartus) use the CD28 co-stimulatory domain. Complete responses to treatment range between 50% and 80%, depending on the product and the injected dose, which varies from 2 to 150 million cells.

The B-cell maturation antigen (BCMA) is a protein expressed on the surface of malignant plasma cells. Plasma cells are fully differentiated B cells that produce and secrete large quantities of antibodies specific to a particular antigen. They are typically long-lived and do not proliferate. BCMA-targeted CAR-T cells have been approved for relapsed/refractory multiple myeloma. The BCMA–CAR-T cell products *idecabtagene vicleucel* (Abecma) and *ciltacabtagene autoleucel* (Carvykti) use 4-1BB as co-stimulatory domain. Complete response is observed between 25% and 40% of patients depending on the dose for Abecma and 83% for Carvykti. While Abecma uses a dosage of 150–450 million cells, Carvykti uses 0.75 million cells. Thus, Carvykti seems to demonstrate superior efficacy at a lower dose.

Some explanations can be given about the differences between Abecma and Carvytki. While both therapies are used for multiple myeloma, Abecma is typically administered after more prior lines of therapy compared to Carvykti, which can be given earlier in the treatment process. This could explain the higher success ratio of Carvykti.

Indeed, Abecma is approved for the treatment of adult patients with relapsed or refractory multiple myeloma who have received at least two prior lines of therapy, including a proteasome inhibitor, an immunomodulatory agent, and an anti-CD38 monoclonal antibody. In the KarMMA trial, Abecma showed overall and complete response rates of 73% and 33%, respectively. On the other end, Carvykti is approved for the treatment of adult patients with relapsed or refractory multiple myeloma who have received at least one prior line of therapy, including a proteasome inhibitor and an immunomodulatory agent, and are refractory to lenalidomide. In the Cartitude 1 study, Carvykti showed responses in 98% of participants, with 78% achieving a complete response.

As mentioned in Section 8.6, CAR-T cell engineering necessitates stable transduction or transfection, which means chromosomal integration of the CAR gene into a large number of T lymphocytes. T-cell engineering was initiated using Moloney murine leukemia virus γ-oncoretroviral vectors, and it was later extended to include lentiviral vectors and DNA transposons, all of which mediate stable long-term transgene. Breyanzi, Tecartus, and Yescarta utilize γ-retroviral vectors to deliver specific CARs into T cells. Lentiviral vectors, which are derived from HIV-1 and pseudotyped with the VSV-G envelope, are used for transgene integration into CAR-T cells for Abecma, Carvykti, Kymriah, and JWCAR029.

## 8.8 Tumor Resistance and the Challenge of Solid Tumors

A limitation for CAR-T cell treatment arises from the CD19 down-regulation in a subpopulation of leukemia or lymphoma tumor T cells, which ultimately escape CAR-T cell treatment and lead to relapse. For instance, several 2017–2018 reports indicated that up to 30% of patients who had relapsed after CD19 CAR-T cell therapy had CD19-negative disease. Since there are other markers specific to B cells, such as CD20 and CD22, CARs have been designed against these markers, leading to successful treatment with CAR-T cells in these relapsing patients. More recently, bispecific CD19–CD20 and even trispecific CAR-T cells have shown interesting results in CD19-CAR relapsed patients. One way to produce these divalent or trivalent CAR-T cells is to introduce a construct containing a 2A viral sequence for simultaneous expression of equal concentrations of each CAR at the cell membrane.

In addition, although CAR-T cells have been tremendously successful for treating several of the most severe hematological malignancies, multiple challenges must be overcome in order to generalize their use to solid tumors. Indeed, in 2025, the approved CAR-T cells were restricted to hematopoietic cancers expressing two antigens, CD19 and BCMA. The efficacy of CAR-T cells in treating solid tumors is lagging behind and still needs technological improvements before reaching the clinical stages. The resistance of solid tumors to CAR-T cell treatment results from several factors, among which are the absence or insufficient level of expression of the CAR target in tumor cells (antigen escape), a lack of antigenic homogeneity within solid tumors, low tumor infiltration especially into the ischemic core or solid tumors, and local immune suppression induced in the tumor microenvironment. In addition, in Section 8.9, examples of toxicity linked to off-tumor (off-target) effects are presented, illustrating cases where the selected antigen is also expressed in healthy cells.

The primary problem concerns the identification of suitable target antigens. Several clinical trials or advanced preclinical work involve targeting L1CAM for neuroblastoma, receptor tyrosine kinase-like orphan receptor 1 (ROR1) for triple-negative breast cancer, MUC16 (mucin 16) for primary peritoneal and Fallopian tube cancer, and LeY for advanced solid tumors. Actively investigated targets, among others, include carcinoembryonic antigen (CEA) for various carcinomas, including colon cancer and liver metastasis, and MUC1 (mucin 1) and alpha-fetoprotein for liver cancer.

Although an ScFv moiety in the fusion protein is the most common targeting head in prototype CARs, other ligands have also been proposed.

For instance, the proliferation-inducing ligand APRIL has been fused either as a monomer or as a fusion trimer to target two proteins that are highly expressed on multiple myeloma tumor cells: BCMA and TACI (transmembrane activator and CAML interactor), which are members of the tumor necrosis factor (TNF) receptor superfamily.

A second challenge specific to solid tumors is the poor penetration of CAR-T cells into the tumoral tissue. This is caused not only by a mechanical barrier that hampers T-cell penetration into non-vascularized deep hypoxic tumor zones, but also by a generally immunosuppressive environment linked to hypoxic conditions and the release of anergizing cytokines. A proposed approach to overcome this central limitation is based on co-treatment with small molecules or checkpoint inhibitors, which interfere with the immunosuppressive pathways. A complementary approach has been to load CAR-T cells with an immunostimulatory cytokine gene, such as IL-12, contingent upon the intracellular activation signal in these cells. The immunostimulatory cytokine is then released in the immediate vicinity of the tumor. However, some toxicity has been observed in early clinical trials involving IL-12 CAR-T cells, so special caution should be exercised when using this potentially synergistic strategy.

## 8.9  Toxicity Challenges and Safety Considerations

Although prospects for the treatment of a large variety of tumors are exciting, many challenges remain to be overcome. First, toxicity due to the treatment has been observed, mainly concerning severe cytokine release syndrome (CRS), which can lead to neurotoxicity and, in some cases, death. This toxicity is further increased by the conditioning regimen necessary to deplete the naïve T-cell population in the patient before administering the CAR-T cells. The administration of corticoids and anti-cytokine antibodies, such as anti-IL-6, appears to alleviate most CRS manifestations; however, their use is limited in order to avoid inhibiting CAR-T cells themselves, which is the case with glucocorticoids. Acute CRS toxicity was observed when using the most aggressive third-generation CARs, and the difficulty in handling these tremendously potent CAR-T cells has precluded their further clinical development so far.

Another limitation for the generalization of CAR-T cells is identifying selective targets. Ideally, the target should be present only on the tumor tissue, since off-target effects might lead to severe unwanted damage to a life-essential tissue. For instance, the targeting of epithelial growth factor 2 (EERB2) has been investigated in an advanced colon cancer patient with liver metastases. The patient was treated with an anti-EERB2 second-generation CAR containing a fragment of the humanized monoclonal antibody Herceptin and an optimized costimulatory signal. The patients suffered severe lung inflammation and edema, linked to the fact that EERB2 is also present on lung epithelial cells, which led to CRS and, ultimately, to the patient's death. In another example, patients with metastatic renal carcinoma were treated with a CAR-T cell targeting the renal marker carbonic-anhydrase IX (CAIX). Hepatotoxicity was observed due to the presence of CAIX on biliary epithelium. These two examples stress the necessary caution in selecting an antigen for CAR-T cell therapy.

Solutions have been proposed to alleviate such off-target effects, mainly based on combinatorial antigen recognition. The first strategy consists of making CARs dependent on the simultaneous presence of two antigens, which might be selectively present only on tumor cells. Alternatively, a second strategy is based on the specific presence of a given target on normal cells but not tumor cells and consists of equipping the CAR-T cells with two CARs: an activating CAR recognizing the antigen present on both tumor and normal cells, and an additional inhibitory CAR (iCAR) containing a death signal such as Programmed Death 1 (PD-1) or CTLA4. The role of this iCAR is to attenuate or even suppress any CAR T-cell attacks on normal cells (Figure 8.6).

One way to improve the safety of CAR-T cell treatments is to use a suicide gene approach, allowing for the destruction of CAR-T cells on demand. Ideally, this response should occur within a very short time frame in order to control CRS or GVH syndrome. The first approach involves introducing a gene whose products will kill CAR-T cells upon administration of a chemical drug. Classical suicide genes include the herpes simplex thymidine kinase (HSV-TK) gene or the inducible caspase-9 (iC9) gene, with the latter leading to faster action than HSV-TK. Another

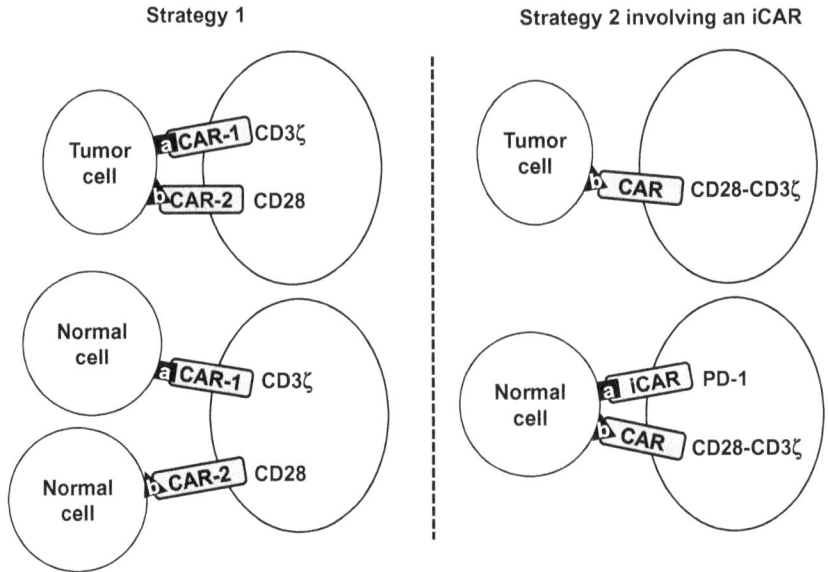

**Figure 8.6.** Proposed strategies to improve CAR-T cell specificity and alleviate off-target effects. In the first strategy (left), the simultaneous presence of two antigens **a** and **b** is necessary to activate both CD33ζ and the costimulatory signal CD28. If only one of the antigens **a** or **b** is present on different normal cells, the CAR-T cell will not kill that cell. In the second strategy (right), the selective presence of antigen **a** on a normal cell triggers the PD-1-mediated signal of the inhibitory iCAR, leading to the death of the CAR-T cell.

elegant approach is to co-transduce T cells with a surface marker, such as the truncated epidermal growth factor receptor (tEGFR). This truncated receptor is devoid of a signal transduction domain but can be targeted by monoclonal antibodies already in clinical use, thus allowing the induction of antibody-dependent cell-mediated cytotoxicity processes against CAR-T cells when necessary.

## 8.10  Perspectives

In conclusion, CAR-T cells represent a revolutionary incremental advance in our fight against cancer, and further significant development of this technology should appear in the future, including the use of other "CAR" cells, such as those obtained by transduction of natural killer (NK) or macrophages, considering the tremendous effort and attention given to adoptive immunotherapy. For instance, NK cells seem to have a higher potency in penetrating tumor cells compared to T-lymphocytes in a neuroblastoma tumor using the anti-ganglioside D2 (GD2) CAR.

Progress should also come from the use of "off-the-shelf" universal heterologous T-cells, thus avoiding the tedious steps involved in obtaining autologous CAR-T cells. This option is particularly appealing because T-cells in patients who have received heavy anticancer drug treatment can become exhausted, leading to low potency of autologous CAR T-cells.

Major progress is expected from precision genome editing techniques, which would allow improving and refining CAR-T cell functions. This has been described, for instance, by ablating CAR-T cell TCR in order to avoid GVH, or by deleting their MHC molecules in order to allow heterologous "universal" CAR-T cells to survive in the host environment without being rejected. Also, CAR-T cells in which the PD-1 immune checkpoint receptor has been deleted exhibit greater tumor cell killing ability, improved immunotherapy efficacy, reduced T-cell exhaustion, and increased memory T-cell capacity; they are being developed at the clinical stage. In the latter case, genome editing was not used; instead, the transduction vector incorporates a short hairpin RNA cassette targeting PD-1 into a BCMA-CAR with an OX-40 costimulatory domain.

Finally, the application of CAR-T cells will, without doubt, be expanded in the future for the treatment of autoimmune, inflammatory, and infectious diseases. For autoimmune and inflammatory diseases, promising preclinical results have been described for the following conditions: systemic lupus erythematosus, rheumatoid arthritis, multiple sclerosis, and myasthenia gravis.

## Bibliography

Abou-El-Enein M, Elsallab M, Feldman SA, *et al*. Scalable Manufacturing of CAR-T cells for Cancer Immunotherapy. *Blood Cancer Discov*. 2021 Sep;2(5):408–22. doi: 10.1158/2643-3230.BCD-21-0084.

Ahmad A, Uddin S, Steinhoff M. CAR-T cell therapies: an overview of clinical studies supporting their approved use against acute lymphoblastic leukemia and large B-cell lymphomas. *Int J Mol Sci.* 2020 May 30;21(11):3906. doi: 10.3390/ijms21113906.

Berdecka D, De Smedt SC, De Vos WH, Braeckmans K. Non-viral delivery of RNA for therapeutic T cell engineering. *Adv Drug Deliv Rev.* 2024 May;208:115215. doi: 10.1016/j.addr.2024.115215.

Billingsley MM, Gong N, Mukalel AJ, Thatte AS, El-Mayta R, Patel SK, Metzloff AE, Swingle KL, *et al. In vivo* mRNA CAR T cell engineering via targeted ionizable lipid nanoparticles with extrahepatic tropism. *Small.* 2024 Mar;20(11):e2304378. doi: 10.1002/smll.202304378.

Erler P, Kurcon T, Cho H, Skinner J, Dixon C, Grudman S, Rozlan S, Dessez E, *et al.* Multi-armored allogeneic MUC1 CAR T cells enhance efficacy and safety in triple-negative breast cancer. *Sci Adv.* 2024 Aug 30;10(35):eadn9857. doi: 10.1126/sciadv.adn9857.

Eshhar Z, Waks T, Gross G. The emergence of T-bodies/CAR T cells. *Cancer J.* 2014 Mar-Apr;20(2):123–6. doi: 10.1097/PPO.0000000000000027.

Garfall AL, Stadtmauer EA, Hwang WT, Lacey SF, Melenhorst JJ, Krevvata M, Carroll MP, Matsui WH, *et al.* Anti-CD19 CAR T cells with high-dose melphalan and autologous stem cell transplantation for refractory multiple myeloma. *JCI Insight.* 2018 Apr 19;3(8):e120505. doi: 10.1172/jci.insight.120505.

Globerson Levin A, Rivière I, Eshhar Z, Sadelain M. CAR T cells: building on the CD19 paradigm. *Eur J Immunol.* 2021 Sep;51(9):2151–63. doi: 10.1002/eji.202049064.

Heczey A, Xu X, Courtney AN, Tian G, Barragan GA, Guo L, Amador CM, Ghatwai N, Rathi P, *et al.* Anti-GD2 CAR-NKT cells in relapsed or refractory neuroblastoma: updated phase 1 trial interim results. *Nat Med.* 2023 Jun;29(6):1379–88. doi: 10.1038/s41591-023-02363-y.

June CH, O'Connor RS, Kawalekar OU, Ghassemi S, Milone MC. CAR T cell immunotherapy for human cancer. *Science.* 2018 Mar 23;359(6382):1361–5. doi: 10.1126/science.aar6711.

Köhler M, Greil C, Hudecek M, Lonial S, Raje N, Wäsch R, Engelhardt M. Current developments in immunotherapy in the treatment of multiple myeloma. *Cancer.* 2018 May 15;124(10):2075–85. doi: 10.1002/cncr.31243.

Li K, Lan Y, Wang J, *et al.* Chimeric antigen receptor-engineered T cells for liver cancers, progress and obstacles. *Tumour Biol.* 2017 Mar;1–8.

Nguyen NTT, Müller R, Briukhovetska D, Weber J, Feucht J, Künkele A, Hudecek M, Kobold S. The Spectrum of CAR Cellular Effectors: Modes of Action in Anti-Tumor Immunity. *Cancers (Basel).* 2024 Jul 22;16(14):2608. doi: 10.3390/cancers16142608.

Ouyang W, Jin SW, Xu N, Liu WY, Zhao H, Zhang L, Kang L, Tao Y, *et al.* PD-1 downregulation enhances CAR-T cell antitumor efficiency by preserving a cell memory phenotype and reducing exhaustion. *J Immunother Cancer.* 2024 Apr 8;12(4):e008429. doi: 10.1136/jitc-2023-008429.

Rasche L, Hudecek M, Einsele H. CAR T-cell therapy in multiple myeloma: mission accomplished? *Blood.* 2024 Jan 25;143(4):305–10. doi: 10.1182/blood.2023021221.

Rurik JG, Tombácz I, Yadegari A, Méndez Fernández PO, Shewale SV, Li L, Kimura T, Soliman OY, Papp TE, *et al.* CAR T cells produced in vivo to treat cardiac injury. *Science.* 2022 Jan 7;375(6576):91–6. doi: 10.1126/science.abm0594.

Sadelain M, Rivière I, Riddell S. Therapeutic T cell engineering. *Nature.* 2017 May 24;545(7655):423–31. doi: 10.1038/nature22395.

Short L, Holt RA, Cullis PR, *et al.* Direct in vivo CAR T cell engineering. *Trends Pharmacol Sci.* 2024 May;45(5):406–18. doi: 10.1016/j.tips.2024.03.004.

Srivastava S, Tyagi A, Pawar VA, Khan NH, Arora K, Verma C, Kumar V. Revolutionizing Immunotherapy: Unveiling New Horizons, Confronting Challenges, and Navigating Therapeutic Frontiers in CAR-T Cell-Based Gene Therapies. *Immunotargets Ther.* 2024 Aug 27;13:413–33. doi: 10.2147/ITT.S474659.

Wang H, Kadlecek TA, Au-Yeung BB, Sjölin Goodfellow HE, Hsu LY, Freedman TS, Weiss A. ZAP-70: An Essential Kinase in T-cell Signaling. *Cold Spring Harb Perspect Biol.* 2010. doi: 10.1101/cshperspect.a002279.

# Chapter 9

# Gene, Base, and Prime Editing

## 9.1 Introduction

New-generation sequencing has opened access to whole-genome determination for every patient when needed. This allows to envision revolutionary personalized medicine, where genetic mutations might be identified and corrected at the individual level. Targeted gene modification via homologous recombination (HR) represents the key necessary tool for these exciting personalized genetic corrections.

HR is a type of genetic recombination where genetic material is exchanged between two DNA molecules carrying similar or identical sequences. This process is crucial for several biological functions. It helps repair harmful breaks in DNA, particularly double-strand breaks, ensuring the integrity of the genetic material. During meiosis, HR produces new combinations of DNA sequences, contributing to genetic variation in offspring. Finally, in bacteria and viruses, HR facilitates the exchange of genetic material between different strains or species, which can spread traits such as antibiotic resistance.

For a gene therapy prospect, HR can be used to insert a DNA sequence into a chromosome. A DNA sequence that is homologous to the target site on the chromosome is designed. This sequence includes the desired DNA to be inserted. The cell's natural HR machinery recognizes the homologous regions and facilitates the exchange of genetic material, integrating the new DNA sequence into the chromosome at the target site. Ideally, this can lead to the correction of a genetic defect, such as a stop codon mutation which induces the synthesis of a non-functional protein.

Genome engineering, which means the capacity to delete, insert, and modify genomic DNA sequences in cells or organisms, encompasses a much wider range of applications compared to personalized gene therapy, covering fields as wide ranging as functional genomics (allowing the study of the function of DNA sequences in their endogenous genomic site), cell line modification, the generation of knock-out or knock-in transgenic animal models by template injection into fertilized eggs, and the optimization of recombinant microorganisms for biotechnological applications, including crop production and fermenter bioproduction. Two classes of techniques have emerged for targeted genome modification, using either protein-based or, more recently, RNA-based recognition of the targeted genomic DNA sequences.

## 9.2 Protein-Based DNA Targeting by Meganucleases and TALEN

Nuclease-mediated targeted genetic correction technology is based on non-homologous end-joining (NHEJ), HR, homologous direct repair (HDR), and the different techniques initially used for specifically modifying the genome of living cells. These techniques require the use of protein nucleases bearing specific DNA-recognition properties, such as meganuclease, zinc-finger nucleases, or TALENs, which allow an efficient modification of various eukaryotic cells.

All these early approaches use customized protein domains for sequence-specific DNA binding. The meganucleases integrate their nuclease and DNA-binding domains into the same protein module and are obtained through molecular evolution and selection. Conversely, zinc-finger nucleases and TALEN technologies use a building block "lexicon" consisting of protein domains which recognize specific DNA sequences. In the Cys2-His2 zinc-finger nucleases, each protein domain recognizes three DNA base pairs, while in TALENs, each domain is specific to a single base pair. These protein domains are then assembled linearly in order to target specific 18 base-pair DNA sequences on the genome and are linked to a FOKI endonuclease moiety.

An additional, customized, protein-based DNA-targeting system, described in Figure 9.1, has been developed more recently. It involves a recombinase-mediated step analogous to the Cre/loxP system. The Cre recombinase is an enzyme derived from the P1 bacteriophage, and the loxP sequence is a 34 base-pairs specific DNA sequence recognized by the enzyme Cre recombinase for site-specific recombination. In the modified system presented here, the Cre recombinase has been optimized by

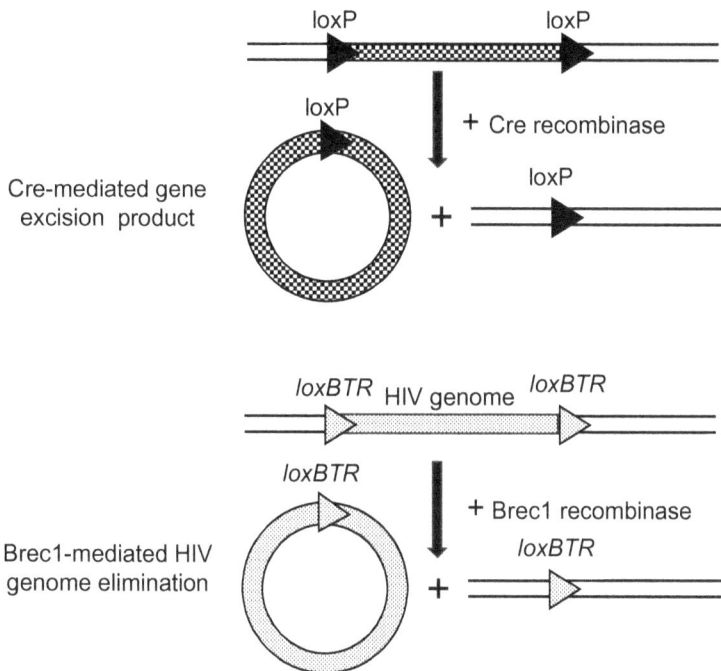

**Figure 9.1.** Mechanism of sequence excision from a prokaryotic genome by the classically used Cre/loxP system and the Brec1 recombinase. The Cre recombinase excises the sequence located between two loxP sites. The Brec1 recombinase has been optimized through molecular evolution and subsequent rationale structure-based modifications in order to recognize the loxBTR sequences present in the genomes of a large number of HIV-1 subtypes and variants.

selection-directed molecular evolution and involved further structure-aided computational optimization in order to bind and recombine a sequence present on a large proportion of HIV-1 strains, which is called loxBTR. The obtained Brec1 recombinase is able to excise an integrated HIV-1 genome from infected cells. Such an elegant genome engineering approach potentially enables us to "cure" HIV-1-infected cells by excising the integrated HIV-1 genomes through gene transfer of the Brec1 recombinase.

## 9.3   RNA-Guided CRISPR/Cas9 DNA Endonuclease: A Bacterial Acquired Immunity System

The above protein-based genome-editing technologies are time-consuming and, in some instances, show low efficacy; moreover, certain particular limitations arise in the cases of TALENs and zinc-finger nucleases due to undesired intramolecular interaction between the adjacent modular motifs used to target genomic sequences. A very efficient, fast-developing genome-editing technology has been introduced since 2013: CRISPR/Cas9, which makes use of an RNA guide capable of locating the endonuclease Cas9 to a specific genomic locus in both prokaryotic and eukaryotic cells. The CRISPR/Cas system has been elucidated through years of fundamental research and represents a remarkable system of microbial "acquired immunity," which was surprising, given that the adaptive immune response is widely considered to be a specific prerogative of multicellular eukaryotic species.

The abbreviation "CRISPR" stands for: clustered regularly interspaced short palindromic repeats. These CRISPR direct repeats had been observed several years before CRISPR/Cas9 discovery in a high proportion of bacterial genomes; however, their significance had remained mysterious. It was then discovered that the "SPACERS" genomic sequences, which are inserted between the CRISPR direct repeats, originate from the genomes of various bacteriophages, which are bacteria-infecting viruses. When a bacteriophage sequence is inserted into the CRISPR array, the bacteria become resistant to the bacteriophage. Thus, the bacterial CRISPR/SPACER array is used as an immune memory and defense system by a wide range of bacteria.

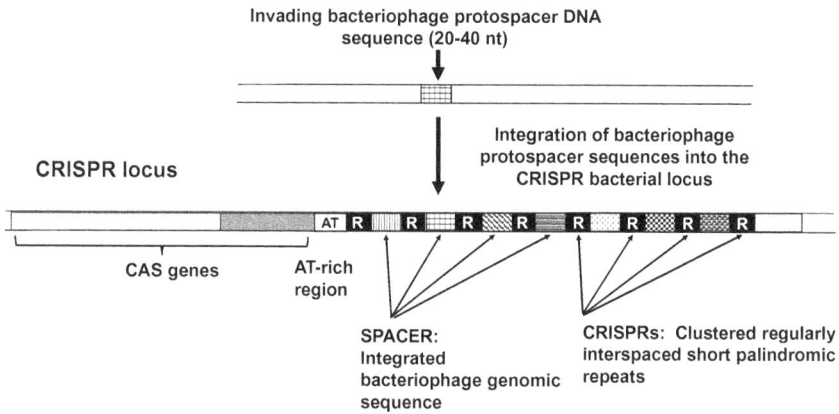

**Figure 9.2.** Bacteriophage protospacer acquisition and insertion as a SPACER into the CRISPR array.

Figure 9.2 describes how a short (20–40) nucleotide (nt) sequence from an invading bacteriophage is cut from the phage genome and inserted into the multiple CRISPR direct-repeat array. The bacteriophage DNA sequences are called "protospacer" sequences. They are cut and inserted as SPACERS into the bacterial CRISPR locus through the action of CRISPR-associated nucleases (Cas nuclease), thus conferring to the bacteria the capacity to become resistant to the phage.

In the following step of the CRISPR defense mechanism, the CRISPR locus is transcribed into a non-coding RNA array, the pre-crRNA (pre-CRISPR-RNA). This long pre-crRNA is matured in a process which varies among the three diverse types of CRISPR systems: types I, II, and III. Each CRISPR type possesses a specific cleavage and process mechanism, but all three types lead to the generation of small crRNAs containing an individual SPACER RNA sequence and a direct-repeat sequence (or part of it). The small crRNAs possess a double function:

- The direct-repeat sequence is able to bind and modulate the properties of a set of Cas nucleases that are specific for each CRISPR type.
- The SPACER RNA sequence is used as an invading RNA strand, which hybridizes (i.e., base-pairs) according to Watson–Crick rules with the bacteriophage DNA targeted sequence.

According to this dual function, the SPACER RNA "guides" the Cas nuclease for specific cleavage at a given site in an invading bacteriophage genome. This exquisite targeting property is the cornerstone of the gene-editing and gene therapy use of the CRISPR defense system.

While the type I and type III CRISPR systems recruit a complex assembly of several Cas proteins, in contrast, the type II CRISPR system only requires a single endonuclease called Cas9. This simpler type II system is the one used for genome editing in eukaryotic cells, and it will be further described in this chapter. Most progress has been obtained with the CRISPR type II system of Streptococcus pyogenes, which uses the SpCas9 nuclease, and with Streptococcus thermophilus (StCas9).

In type II CRISPR, a bacterial trans-activating CRISPR RNA (tracrRNA) hybridizes with the direct-repeat sequence. Through a mechanism that is not completely elucidated, involving the RNase III enzyme, a set of RNA duplexes is generated via Watson–Crick base-pairing between a crRNA and a tracrRNA, as shown in Figure 9.3.

The final steps of the type II CRISPR defense mechanism are schematized in Figure 9.4. The crRNA/tracrRNA duplex associates with the

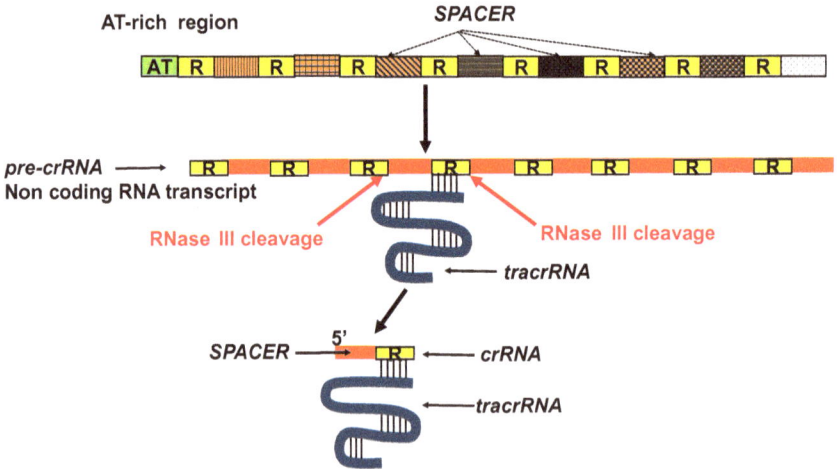

**Figure 9.3.**   Annealing of tracrRNA and RNase III cleavage releases a set of RNA duplexes with bacteriophage targeting capacity.

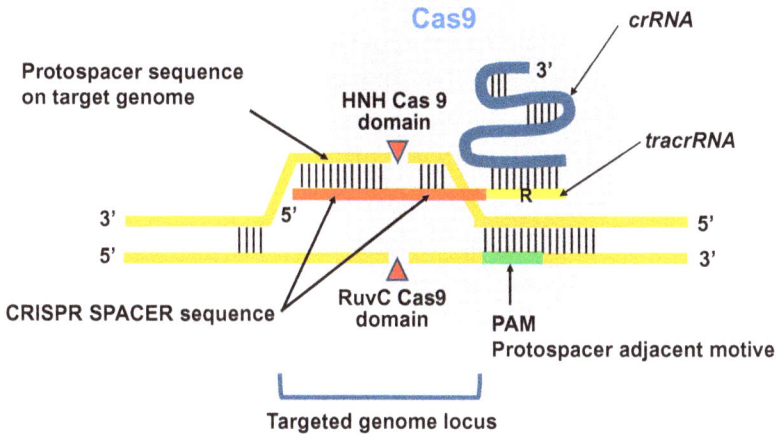

**Figure 9.4.** Loading of the crRNA/tracrRNA duplex onto the Cas9 nuclease is followed by recognition of the PAM on the bacteriophage genome, then by invasion and hybridization of the phage DNA by the SPACER RNA, and finally by phage genome nucleolytic cleavage by the Cas9 active sites RuvC and HNH (red arrowheads). Binding to bacteriophage genomic DNA requires that the protospacer sequence of the targeted genomic locus perfectly match that of the SPACER region of the gRNA, and it must have a PAM next to the protospacer. The Cas9 protein contains two nuclease domains, HNH and RuvC. The HNH domain is responsible for cleaving the DNA strand which is complementary to the guide RNA (the target strand), while the RuvC domain cleaves the non-target strand.

Cas9 nuclease by binding to its positively charged groove. The resulting ternary RNA/RNA/protein ribonucleoprotein complex then scouts the bacteriophage DNA and binds weakly to a genetic motif adjacent to the bacteriophage protospacer sequence, called the "protospacer adjacent motif (PAM)". This weak binding allows the 20 nt SPACER sequence of the crRNA/tracrRNA duplex to invade the bacteriophage DNA and hybridize into with the bacteriophage protospacer. This annealing then leads to a Cas9 conformational change, which activates the nuclease activity and leads to double-strand cleavage of the bacteriophage DNA by Cas9.

The double-strand break occurs through the action of two Cas9 enzymatic active sites: RuvC and HNH. This last step ultimately leads to phage elimination and confers bacterial resistance. The RuvC Cas9 catalytic site cleaves the DNA strand bearing the PAM, while the HNH site cuts the phage DNA strand that is complementary to the crRNA guide. The cleavage occurs about 3–4 nt upstream of the PAM sequence.

It is worth mentioning that once the ribonucleoprotein CRISPR complex binds to the PAM site, the protospacer strand invasion begins through a seed sequence located 8–10 bases at the 3' end of the gRNA SPACER sequence. Only if the seed annealing shows a perfect match will the gRNA continue to anneal in the 3'–5' direction via zipper-like cooperative Watson–Crick hybridization. In contrast to the first "seed" annealing process, the latter cooperative process might occur even in the presence of a slight mismatch, which thus induces an "off target" double-strand break. As will be described later, several strategies have been proposed to decrease off-target cleavage, thereby improving the biosafety of the CRISPR/Cas9 system in genome editing and gene therapy applications.

Several key features are necessary to the efficiency and safety of the CRISPR immune defense process within bacteria. First, the Cas9 nuclease alone (apoCas9) is naturally inactive and is only activated when bound to both the PAM and the targeted protospacer sequence present on the bacteriophage DNA, as shown in Figure 9.4. Second, the direct repeats of the CRISPR locus are devoid of PAMs, which prevents the CRISPR locus from being "self" auto-attacked by the ribonucleoprotein complex.

## 9.4 Improvement and Simplification of CRISPR/Cas9 System

As soon as it was discovered that the CRISPR/Cas9 ribonucleoprotein complex could be efficiently transplanted and activated in eukaryotic cells, the gene-editing capacity of this simple yet versatile system appeared tremendously promising. Indeed, instead of having to reconstruct *de novo* an entire protein for every targeted sequence, the CRISPR/Cas9 system only requires an appropriate RNA guide containing a SPACER sequence complementary to the targeted genomic site. The main remaining condition to fulfill is that a convenient PAM should be located in the vicinity of this targeted genomic site. In contrast to other gene-editing systems (TALENs, zinc-finger nucleases, etc.), the tool that is only required is a proper and specific RNA guide, which must be synthesized or constructed within a plasmid and associated with a generic Cas9 nuclease.

In order to further simplify this platform, the crRNA/tracrRNA duplex described above in Figure 9.4 is now most frequently replaced by a single-stranded guiding RNA (single guide RNA, sgRNA) covering the dual functions of the duplex, as shown in Figure 9.5. Since the targeting annealing moiety of the sgRNA is about 20 nt long, the use of several RNA guides in the same cell opens the way to parallel multiplex editing in several genomic loci, thus expanding the perspectives of the technology for genome functional screening and multiple genetic correction. In consequence, the CRISPR/Cas9 system has rapidly become the major technique currently used for gene-targeting applications.

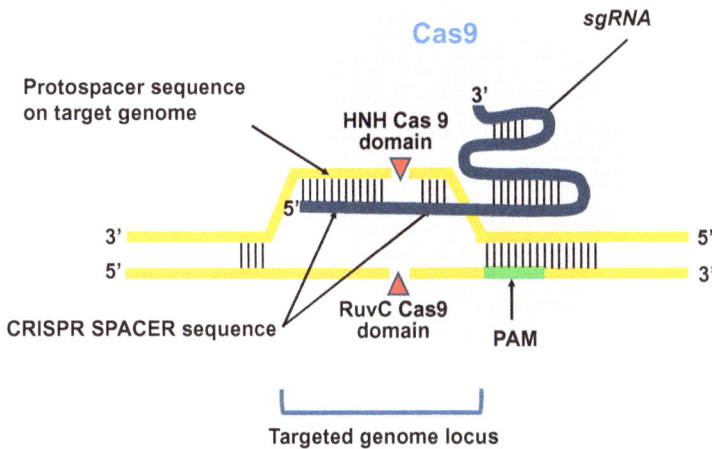

**Figure 9.5.** The CRISPR/Cas9 single guide RNA (sgRNA) system. The nuclease Cas9 first complexes with sgRNA, which comprises a 20-nt-long SPACER region at the 5' end and an 80-nt-long backbone at the 3' end. Binding to genomic DNA requires that the protospacer sequence of the targeted genomic locus be perfectly complementary to that of the SPACER region of the gRNA and contain a protospacer-adjacent-motif (PAM) next to the protospacer. After the Cas9:sgRNA ribonucleoprotein complex binds to the genomic locus of interest, Cas9 undergoes a conformational change that activates its double nuclease activity in the RuvC and HNH domains. The HNH domain is responsible for cleaving the DNA strand that is complementary to the guide RNA (the target strand), while the RuvC domain cleaves the non-target strand. This produces a double-strand break (DSB) at the required locus, leading to either non-homologous end joining or HR, as described in Figure 9.6.

Gene editing might have two aims. The first one is the inactivation of a pathologic gene, such as an oncogene, an infectious genome, or any dominant negative gene. After a double-strand break, the natural cellular repair process involves non-homologous end joining NHEJ, which causes numerous non-specific small insertion or deletion events (indel) (Figure 9.6). Thus, repetitive NHEJ naturally leads to gene inactivation. This mechanism is used in most of the gene-editing clinical applications to date. The situation is different if the DSB occurs while a DNA template is introduced, which bears a sequence homology with both sides of the DSB. In such a case, the sequence between the 5' and 3' homology fragments is inserted into the DSB. Thus, it becomes possible to correct a dominant negative mutation by inserting the "healthy" wild-type sequence between the two homologous strands of the template. Such a process is commonly used to either repair a defect (homology-directed gene repair) or to introduce a desired sequence at a defined genomic locus (Figure 9.6).

The PAM necessary for the initial binding of the ribonucleoprotein complex is specific in each Cas nuclease ortholog from different bacterial strains. For instance, the Streptococcus pyogenes SpCas9 PAM sequence is 5' NGG, a degenerated recognition codon which allows the CRISPR

**Cas 9 induced double strand break**

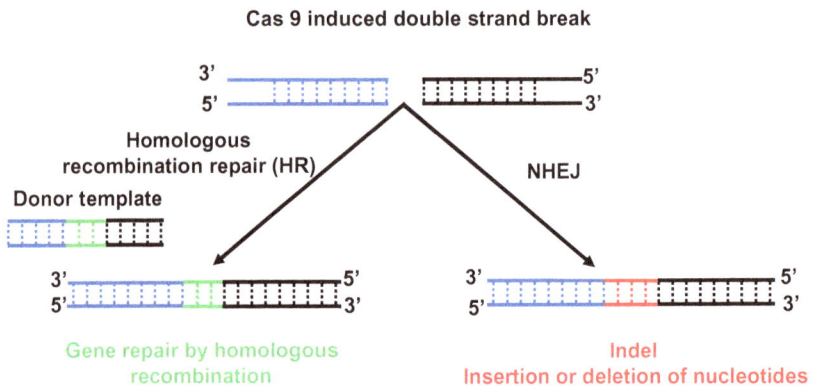

**Figure 9.6.** Mechanism of gene editing following a double-strand break mediated by the CRISPR/Cas9 system. NHEJ introduces non-specific indels, which might inactivate the gene. The addition of a homologous template allows for the repair of a defective gene or the insertion of a desired sequence at a defined genomic locus. Gene editing through meganuclease or TALEN-induced double-strand breaks follows the same mechanism.

ribonucleoprotein complex to bind on average to every 8 bp in a human genome. This confers a large but incomplete targeting capacity for gene editing and thus restricts the versatility of the technology. Such a limitation represents an important concern for HR, which requires very precise double-strand break locations. To circumvent this problem, other Cas9 nucleases requiring a different PAM sequence have been made available, such as the following:

- Streptococcus thermophilus StCas9 (PAM: 3' NNAGAAW),
- acidaminococcus sp. AsCpf1 (PAM: 5' TTTV),
- lachnospiraceae bacterium LbCpf1 (PAM: 5' TTTV),
- or Staphylococcus aureus (PAM: 3' NNGRRT or NNGRR(N)).

In addition, mutated variants of SpCas9, AsCpf1, and LbCpf1 have been identified with different PAM sequences. Overall, the diversity of PAMs recognized by different Cas9 or other Cas orthologs greatly expands the targeting capacity of the CRISPR/Cas system to virtually any targeted site in eukaryotic genomes.

As mentioned above, most applications make use of the nuclease activity of the Cas enzymes to generate double-strand breakage either for either gene inactivation through NHEJ or for gene repair or gene insertion through HR (also called HDR). However, other applications have been developed which only make use of the genome-targeting capacity of the ribonucleoprotein system, such as base editing described as follows. Adequate domains of the Cas nucleases have been modified, for instance by eliminating the Mg++ binding sites necessary for the nuclease activity, and it has been possible to generate mutant ribonucleoprotein complexes with maintained DNA targeting efficiency but devoid of nuclease activity. The RuvC catalytic domain is composed of three parts of the Cas9 protein: RuvC-I near the N-terminal region, and RuvC-II and -III adjacent to the second HNH catalytic sequence near the middle of the protein. The D10A (aspartate => Ala) mutation in RuvC-I inactivates the RuvC's catalytic activity, and the H840A (histidine => Ala) substitution inactivates the HNH second nuclease domain of Cas9. The double mutant, whose nuclease activity is completely inactivated (called "nuclease dead" dCas9), has been fused to a transcriptional activator (such as VP64 or VPR) or repressor (such as KRAB) in order to obtain targeted gene activation or repression, respectively. Other cell biology applications include the fusion of dCas9 with a fluorescent protein, such as green fluorescent protein (GFP), which allows monitoring *in cellulo* the spatial dynamics of a given genomic locus.

The CRISPR single-guide sgRNA is introduced into the cells either as a DNA sequence within a plasmid under a polymerase III promoter, such as U6, or as an RNA produced by *in vitro* transcription. The nuclease Cas9 can also be introduced as a gene under the dependency of a ubiquitous constitutive promoter such as the cytomegalovirus (CMV) promoter. When the Cas nuclease and sgRNA genetic sequences are inserted into a plasmid, they are delivered by classical transfection techniques using chemical vectors (cationic lipids or polymers) or physical delivery techniques (electrotransfer, nucleofection, sonoporation, hydrodynamic delivery, etc.), which are described in Chapters 6 and 7. For cells difficult to transfect or for some *in vivo* applications, recombinant delivery viruses have been developed, primarily involving lentivirus and AAV. However, the cDNA size of the commonly used SpCas9 (about 4 kb) is too large for proper encapsidation into an AAV particle. For this specific application, Staphylococcus aureus Cas9, whose gene is about 3 kb, represents a suitable alternative. Finally, non-viral LNPs are being increasingly used to deliver CRISPR sgRNA and Cas9 mRNA, both *in vitro* and *in vivo*, especially to the liver in the latter case. This strategy has the advantage to decrease the duration of Cas9 nuclease presence within the cells, thus preventing off-target effects (see below).

## 9.5  Reducing Off-Target Effects of CRISPR/Cas9

The negative potential of off-target double-strand breaks in the CRISPR/Cas9 system has received immediate consideration. Off-target cleavage might result from the risk of redundancy in the 20 nt targeting sequence, as well as from the fact that the annealing guide RNA accepts a certain degree of mismatch. Several strategies have been proposed to circumvent this limitation.

The first approach is based on the decrease in the nt size of the annealing sgRNA. It has been noted that a truncated sgRNA significantly increases SpCas9 specificity, presumably because mismatches in shorter annealing sequences have a stronger negative effect of the binding and subsequent nuclease efficiency of the ribonucleoprotein complex.

Second, rationally designed mutations have been introduced in SpCas9 in order to generate high-fidelity Cas9 mutants which either possess a lower affinity for the targeted DNA strands or have improved proofreading capacity.

The third strategy aims to limit the presence time of Cas nuclease in the cell. For this purpose, Cas genetic sequences have been inserted under inducible promoters, such as Tet-on.

The fourth option to limit off-target cleavage is to use preassembled CRISPR ribonucleoproteins, obtained through *in vitro* transcribed sgRNA and recombinant Cas9. Such complexes can be directly delivered into the cells either through *ex vivo* electroporation or by association with cationic lipids. This leads to a very transient ribonucleoprotein presence, thus allowing a decrease in off-target double-strand breaks. Alternatively, both CRISPR nd Cas9 can be delivered in lipid nanoparticles LNPs, taking advantage of the mRNA intracellular short half-life.

Another interesting fifth technique involves the use of a self-limiting CRISPR/Cas9 system to reduce the duration of SpCas9 expression. In this improved system, recognition sites for the sgRNA are introduced into the SpCas9 sequence itself, thus allowing the SpCas9 gene to be excised and eliminated following the intracellular expression of the SpCas9 protein. As a result, the continuous expression of SpCas9 is abolished, and its cellular residence time is limited by protein cellular turnover, which increases biosecurity by decreasing the occurrence of off-target double-strand breaks.

Finally, a very elegant last approach uses Cas9 variants which have been inactivated in either the RuvC (D10A mutation) or the HNH (H840A mutation) catalytic domains. These mutants have lost their capacity to generate double-strand breaks but still retain a nickase activity (i.e., cutting a single strand). Figure 9.7 shows how two Cas9-derived nickases within a CRISPR complex can be used to increase selectivity. In this configuration, a double-strand break will only occur if the two Cas9 nickases are

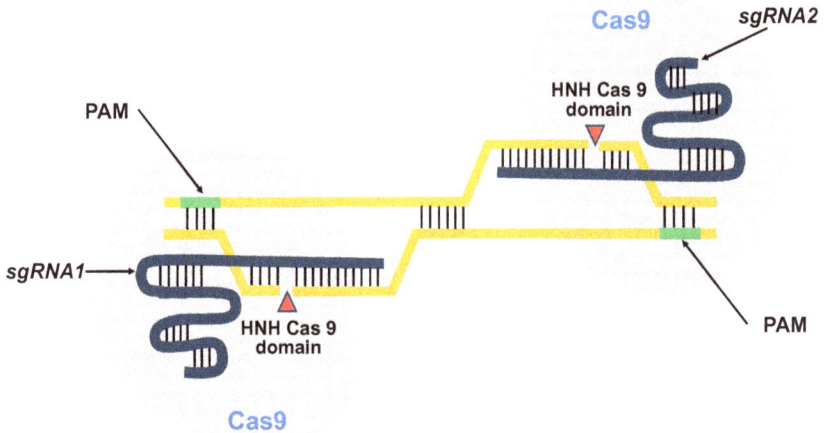

**Figure 9.7.**  Use of two Cas9-derived nickases for highly selective double-strand break targeting with limited off-target effect. In the shown configuration, a D10A-mutated RuvC domain has been introduced into the SpCas9 nuclease.

properly located at proximal genomic sites by two different sgRNA targeting genomic sequences. The probability of two mismatches occurring simultaneously on these two targeted 20 nt sequences is greatly reduced.

## 9.6  Base Editing Without DNA Cleavage

A final, exciting illustration and extension of the CRISPR/Cas9 system application concerns single-base editing. Before the introduction of CRISPR/Cas9, correcting a single-base mutation required double-strand DNA breaks and the use of donor templates in order to repair the DNA through homology-directed repair. Frequent undesired insertions/deletions (indels) result from this approach, and CRISPR/Cas9 base editors represent an exciting, potentially superior, alternative.

Base editing enables the direct conversion of a single mutation base pair, thus allowing restoration of a wild-type gene. The most commonly used base editors currently use a modified CRISPR/Cas9 system. In brief, these base editors comprise a CRISPR/Cas9 inactivated mutant that cannot induce double-strand breaks but maintains a "nickase" single-strand breakage capacity. In base editing, the RuvC domain of the Cas9 protein is typically inactivated. The Cas9 protein is fused to an enzyme which allows single-base conversion in the single-stranded DNA bubble created by Cas9. The opposite strand is then cleaved by the nickase, and DNA repair enzymes insert the corresponding base in front of the edited base, thus leading to the complete and irreversible conversion of a single-mutation sequence into a "wild-type" corrected sequence.

Several single-base editing enzymes have been introduced. Cytosine base editors convert a cytosine (C) to a thymine (T) in the DNA sequence, and adenine base editors convert an adenine (A) to a guanine (G) in the DNA sequence. These base editors convert a purine into the other one, as well as a pyrimidine into the other one. In the first version, a single-stranded specific cytidine deaminase has been used to convert C to uracil within the DNA bubble on the DNA strand complementary to the single CRISPR guide RNA. The system is completed by a uracil glycosylase inhibitor that impedes uracil excision. The nickase activity then nicks the non-edited DNA strand and mobilizes cellular DNA repair processes which replace the G contained in the DNA strand with an A-containing complementary strand. This combination leads to efficient and permanent C•G to T•A base pair conversions in several prokaryotic and eukaryotic cell types, including human embryonic cells (Figure 9.8). A simplified scheme of the complicated process of the C•G to T•A base pair conversion is represented in Figure 9.9. The genomic editing toolkit has been completed with the introduction of an adenosine-deaminase selected by molecular evolution, which allows the A•T to G•C conversion.

More recent reports have described the A•T to C•G transversion, where the term "transversion" can mean either purine to pyrimidine or pyrimidine to purine conversion. This was obtained by using the fusion of mouse alkyladenine DNA glycosylase with nickase Cas9 and deaminase TadA-8e. Laboratory evolution of mouse alkyladenine DNA glycosylase significantly increased A-to-C/T conversion efficiency by up to 73%. In an independent report, an adenine transversion base editor, AYBE (A-to-C and A-to-T) active in mammalian cells, was obtained by fusing an adenine base editor with hypoxanthine excision protein N-methylpurine DNA

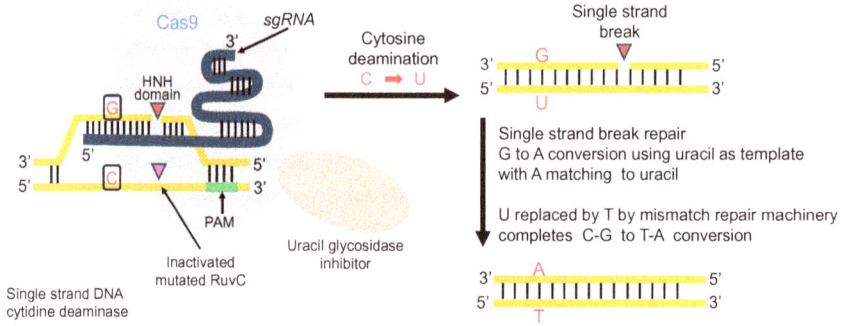

**Figure 9.8.**   C•G to T•A conversion. The RuvC Cas9 domain nuclease activity is inactivated by the D10A mutation, leading to a single-strand break. A single-stranded DNA cytidine deaminase is fused with Cas9 and replaces cytosine with uracil. A uracil-glycosidase protein inhibitor is also fused to Cas9 in order to maintain uracil as a template for replacing G with A during single-strand break repair.

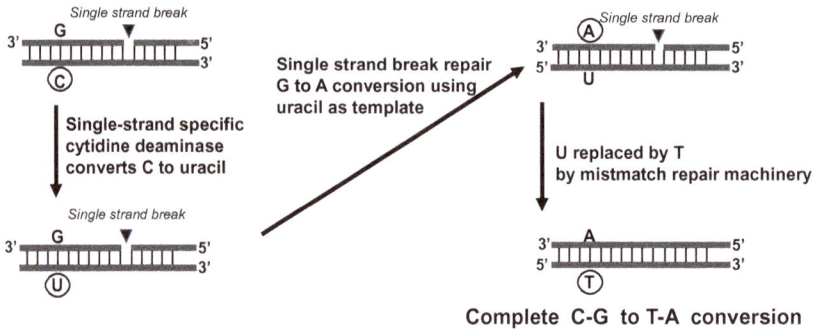

**Figure 9.9.**   Schematic representation of C•G to T•A base pair conversion.

glycosylase, with a high transversion editing activity (up to 72% for A-to-C or A-to-T editing). Base editing progress is striking. In 2025, a first baby was cured from an ultra-rare disease, resulting from a single base mutation in the carbamoyl-phosphate synthetase gene. The carbamoyl-phosphate synthetase (CPS1) enzyme is primarily found in the liver, specifically within hepatocytes, where it plays a crucial role in the urea cycle. A LNP formulation delivered i.v. to the liver was able to drastically decrease ammonemia, which relates to the presence of ammonium ion in the blood, and alleviated most disease symptoms.

## 9.7  Prime Editing

Prime editing represents a more recent genome editing technology than base editing. It aims at directly inserting new genetic information into a specified DNA site using a catalytically impaired Cas9 endonuclease, fused to an engineered reverse transcriptase. The Cas9 endonuclease has been modified to possess a single-strand nickase activity. The reverse transcriptase template is an RNA sequence added to the 3' end of the guide RNA. This modified RNA is designed as pegRNA, for prime editing guide RNA. It contains a 30 nt extension which is present near the nicked target DNA strand. The pegRNA annealed to the targeted DNA sequence serves as a primer-template complex for reverse transcriptase, which polymerizes the desired sequence onto the nicked target DNA site, as specified by the template encoded in the pegRNA. Cellular DNA repair then completes the edited DNA to the genomic DNA. This ideally allows any single base-to-base change, whether a conversion or a transversion. It also allows inserting a desired edit sequence with reasonable efficiency, without needing to involve the homologous recombination repair machinery.

Prime editing has the theoretical potential to correct a large majority of known genetic variants associated with human diseases. It represents a versatile, potent new technique that avoids the risks associated with double-strand breaks. Targeted insertions, deletions, and all twelve types of point mutations, without requiring double-strand breaks or donor DNA templates, have been described using this technology. In addition, prime editing has been shown to induce lower off-target editing than that induced by Cas9-mediated double-strand breaks.

## 9.8  Examples of Genome Editing Therapeutic Applications

A large panel of potential therapeutic applications of CRISPR/Cas9 and other targeted nucleases is being clinically developed or investigated, including, among others, several genetic or infectious diseases affecting the liver, central nervous system (CNS), retina, or muscle. At the end of

2023, an analysis of gene-editing clinical trials in human volunteers by disease type yielded the following numbers: 31 in cancer, 15 for inherited blood disorders (sickle cell and beta-thalassemia), 4 for other inherited disease such as transthyretin amyloidosis, and 2 for fighting viral infections.

**Sickle cell disease and beta-thalassemia:** The first genome editing drug which has been approved by the FDA in December 2023 is *exagamglogene autotemcel* (Casgevy), also known as Exa-cel, to treat sickle cell disease (SCD) in patients aged twelve years and above. This drug uses CRISPR/Cas9 genome-editing technology *ex vivo* to modify patients' hematopoietic (blood) stem cells. The key target is the BCL11A gene, which normally suppresses after birth the expression of fetal hemoglobin HbF, a type of hemoglobin that facilitates oxygen delivery production in the fetus. Casgevy reduces by gene disruption the expression of BCL11A in erythroid lineage cells (the cells that develop into red blood cells), which allows for the reactivation of HbF production. The modified blood stem cells are then transplanted back into the patient, where they engraft (attach and multiply) within the bone marrow and increase HbF production. In patients with sickle cell disease, increased levels of HbF prevent the sickling of red blood cells. This new treatment marked a significant advancement in the field of gene therapy, signaling an innovative progression in the treatment of sickle cell disease. Casgevy is also under the approval procedure for beta-thalassemia. Because HbF can compensate for the lack of normal adult hemoglobin, modified stem cells can raise red blood cell levels in patients with beta-thalassemia.

It has to be noted that genome editing is not the only gene therapy approved for the treatment of sickle cell disease. *Lovotibeglogene autotemcel* (Lyfgenia, lovo-cel) is another gene therapy solution, which was introduced simultaneously. Unlike Casgevy, Lyfgenia uses a lentiviral vector to stably insert the gene HbAT87Q into the chromosomes of hematopoietic stem cells. The gene of HbAT87Q, a variant of hemoglobin A, displays functions similar to that of hemoglobin A. Lyfgenia is approved for the treatment of patients aged 12 years or more with sickle cell disease and a history of vaso-occlusive events.

**Transthyretin amyloidosis:** One notable trial involves the gene-editing therapy NTLA-2001 targeting transthyretin (TTR). TTR amyloidosis, also known as ATTR amyloidosis, is caused by the misfolding of the trans-thyretin protein, a thyroxine and retinol transport protein. Mutant TTR deposition leads to familial TTR amyloid. TTR is a tetramer synthesized by the liver, and genetic mutations induce protein misfolding and the formation of pathological amyloid fibrils in the peripheral nerves and heart, causing polyneuropathy or cardiomyopathy. There have been promising developments in the clinical trials for transthyretin amyloidosis (ATTR) using CRISPR/Cas9-targeted gene inactivation in patients with early genetic ATTR. A transthyretin-targeting CRISPR/Cas9 was delivered IV by a lipid nanoparticle system (LNP; see Chapter 6). Following a single administration, NTLA-2001 resulted in significant editing of the mouse TTR gene and a 96% reduction in serum TTR levels, which lasted for at least 12 months. In the phase 1 trial, patients with ATTR amyloid cardio-myopathy received a single intravenous infusion of NTLA-2001. The results showed a significant reduction in serum TTR levels, by approximately 90%, indicating the therapy's potential to treat this progressive and often-fatal condition.

**Hypercholesterolemia:** It has been noted that naturally occurring loss-of-function of the PCSK9 gene induces a reduction in blood low-density lipoprotein and cholesterol levels. It can be expected from this that PCSK9 gene disruption could confer protection against cardiovascular disease. By using an adenoviral vector to deliver a PCSK9-targeted CRISPR/Cas9 system, a study in mice reported a mutagenesis rate of PCSK9 greater than 50% in the liver. This resulted in decreased blood plasma cholesterol levels by 35–40%. Another application of CRISPR/Cas9 base editing was proposed for preventing cardiovascular risk. As for the PCSK9 gene, it was found that naturally occurring loss-of-function mutations in angiopoietin-like 3 (ANGPTL3) had a beneficial cardiovascular effect, being associated with reduced blood triglycerides and low-density lipoprotein cholesterol, and thus decreasing the risk of coronary heart disease. Two studies have reported that CRISPR/Cas9 base editing of both PCSK9 and ANGPTL3 induces the inactivation of each of these two proteins and that this effect can be obtained *in vivo* in mice. Adenovirus vectors carrying the CRISPR/Cas9 editing system were IV administered, and up to a 35% editing rate was observed in the livers of treated mice. A markedly reduced level of triglycerides and cholesterol was observed in hyperlipidemic mice. This opens the way to *in vivo* base editing to treat patients with atherogenic dyslipidemia. In addition to adenoviral delivery, the use of LNPs has been shown to have a high efficiency for these liver-targeted gene- and base-editing applications.

**Targeted transcriptional activation:** Independently of the potency to correct a mutation through homologous recombination or to inactivate a gene by indels induction following double-strand break and non-homologous end-joining, the capacity of single-guide RNA to target a precise genomic localization can be used to "reactivate" a silent gene or increase a given protein expression. The system comprises an sgRNA that allows targeting a specific genomic site associated with an inactivated Cas9 endonuclease. This deadCas9 (dCas9) is fused to a transcriptional activation domain, for instance the C-terminal VP64 acidic transactivation domain. Multiple therapeutic applications can be envisioned. For instance, utrophin is a fetal muscle protein localized at the muscle fiber (myotube) membrane, whose expression is lost after birth while being replaced by dystrophin. The dystrophin gene is among the largest human genes, and in consequence, its mutations or deletions are responsible for a relatively frequent occurrence of an X-linked genetic disease, Duchenne muscular dystrophy. Attempts to reactivate utrophin expression have been proposed as a treatment for Duchenne muscular dystrophy, and this has been described at the preclinical level in a cellular model by using zinc-finger protein transcription activator-like effectors or CRISPR/Cas9 fused to a transcription activator.

Another application could allow compensating for beta-globin mutations observed in beta-thalassemia and sickle cell anemia by HbF reactivation, potentially leading to the same result as with Casgevy. Friedrich's ataxia is another disease where compensatory reactivation could prove useful since frataxin expression is reduced in cells from Friedreich's ataxia patients due to a trinucleotide repeat expansion in the intron. Finally, CRISPR/Cas9-mediated gene induction has been envisioned for improving the characteristics of cell therapy products in regenerative medicine, for instance to induce the required reprogramming (differentiation and specialization) of pluripotent stem cells.

**Retinal diseases:** Leber congenital amaurosis 10 (LCA10) is a severe retinal dystrophy caused by mutations in the CEP290 gene. The most frequent CEP290 mutation found in human patients is an intronic mutation that generates a cryptic splice donor site. The large size of the CEP290 gene precludes using an adeno-associated virus (AAV) vector for subretinal gene delivery of CEP290, thus eliminating the possibility of gene augmentation therapy, which has been successful in other LCA subtypes (Chapter 3). Hence, other gene therapy solutions have been proposed, such as using an antisense oligonucleotide to mask and thus inactivate the cryptic splice donor site. A study has shown that targeted genomic deletion using CRISPR/Cas9 can suppress this cryptic splice donor in a CEP290 cellular model. Moreover, the study showed the feasibility of introducing *in vivo* precise deletions into retinal cells via subretinal administration of two AAVs: one carrying the sgRNA and the other a SpCAS9 protein.

An additional transcriptional activation potential application is that of age-related muscular degeneration. In its "wet" form, this disease causes loss of vision in a substantial proportion of elderly humans and represents the main cause of blindness among the aging population. About 30% of wet-AMD patients are non-responders to classical anti-VEGF therapy (anti-VEGF monoclonal antibodies, VEGF soluble receptors, or VEGF "traps"). For these patients, the use of pigmented-epithelial derived factor (PEDF) has been proposed. The PEDF represents the most potent identified anti-angiogenic factor, and its targeted transcriptional activation at the vicinity of a retinal macula represents an interesting application of CRISPR-targeted transactivation.

**CAR-T cells base editing:** Base editing has been used to generate universal, off-the-shelf chimeric antigen receptor CAR-T cells (see Chapter 8). Healthy volunteer donor T cells were transduced using a lentivirus to express a CAR with specificity for CD7, a protein expressed in T-cell acute lymphoblastic leukemia (ALL). Base editing has been used to inactivate in these allogenic T cells three genes encoding CD52 and CD7 receptors and the β chain of the αβ T-cell receptor. This has been engineered in order to avoid undesirable side effects of adoptive immunotherapy, which include lymphodepleting serotherapy, CAR7 T-cell fratricide, and graft-versus-host disease, respectively. The safety and efficacy of these edited cells have been reported in three children with relapsed leukemia. However, serious adverse events included cytokine release syndrome, multilineage cytopenia, and opportunistic infections.

**Disruption of integrated HIV genome and HIV receptor CCR5 gene:** Viral diseases, and particularly AIDS, represent one of the most promising therapeutic perspectives of CRISPR/Cas9. While antiretroviral tritherapy effectively controls viremia in HIV-1 patients and partially restores CD4+ T cells to normal levels, this poly-chemotherapy fails to eliminate integrated HIV-1 from latently infected T cells or from other reservoir tissues, such as the CNS. The integrated proviral DNA copies persist in a dormant state and can be reactivated to produce replication-competent viruses, thus re-infecting the patient when drug treatment is stopped. This explains the necessity to develop strategies to effectively "cure" chronically infected T cells and other cell types by a treatment which realizes the excision or disruption of integrated HIV-1 proviral genomes.

There are two intracellular steps in which CRISPR/Cas9 can target the HIV-1 genome and can be used as an intracellular defense against HIV-1: (i) after reverse transcription, and (ii) when the provirus is integrated into the cell chromosomes. In both cases, the double-stranded HIV genome is no longer protected by the viral envelope and capsid, and it is thus prone to nuclease attack. Indeed, efficient CRISPR/Cas9-directed disruption of both infecting HIV-1 viruses and integrated proviruses has been reported *in vitro* in the human embryonic kidney cell line HEK293, several T-cell lines, and human CD4+ T-cells obtained from HIV-1+ patients. In the case of viral disruption, the hypothesis is that intracellular exonucleases further degrade the retro-transcribed HIV genome following CRISPR/Cas9-induced double-strand breaks. In the case of an integrated provirus, mutations, insertions, or deletions (indels) are considered to be the cause of provirus disruption and of the excision of segments of the integrated provirus. Targeting HIV-1 coding regions and the LTR-R region, which contains relatively conserved TAR sequences, is considered a favorable strategy, since the HIV trans-activation response (TAR) element is an RNA element which is required for the trans-activation of the viral promoter and for virus replication. Notably, this excision/disruption process is much more efficient when using a multiplex approach, meaning that multiple gRNA directed against several proviral sequences are necessary in order to achieve significant disruption/excision of the integrated provirus. One of the advantages of the multiplex approach is that it allows circumvention of possible resistance resulting from a mutation occurring in a single sequence targeted by the sgRNA.

These pioneering studies have demonstrated the possibility of generating cells which are self-protected against HIV-1 and even capable of "curing" themselves after HIV-1 infection. Importantly, it has also been shown that engineered human-induced pluripotent stem cells stably expressing HIV-targeted CRISPR/Cas9 could be efficiently differentiated into cell types which are normally HIV reservoirs and that these engineered cells maintain their resistance to HIV-1 infection. Hence, these primary results have opened the way to generating engineered cells possessing acquired protection against HIV-1, which can be self-grafted into patients after modification for personalized gene/cell therapy of HIV-1.

A proof of concept for *in vivo* eradication of HIV-1 in transgenic mice and rats, encompassing the HIV-1 genome, was obtained by delivering RNA-guides/Cas9 through the use of a recombinant adeno-associated virus 9 (rAAV9) vector. Interestingly, AAV9 has been shown to be able to cross the blood–brain barrier (BBB), which is an important clue for treating HIV-1 reservoirs in the CNS. As already mentioned, the smaller Cas9 from Staphylococcus aureus (3.3 kDa) was used here because of the

AAV's limited encapsidation capacity. A multiplex approach was employed, utilizing two sgRNAs to target the LTR1 and Gag sequences. After tail-vein IV administration into mice or after retro-orbital administration into rats, the excision of a 940 bp DNA fragment spanning between the LTR and Gag gene was observed in all tissues (spleen, liver, heart, lung, brain, kidney, and circulating lymphocytes). In addition, the level of viral RNA was drastically reduced (about 80%) in circulating blood cells and lymph nodes of the treated rats. Thus, the multiplex excision with two sgRNA/SaCas9 resulted in a significant decrease in viral transcripts. These encouraging results of *in vivo* HIV-1 partial eradication should pave the way for clinical trials using CRISPR sgRNA/Cas9 in association with classical poly-chemotherapy.

Finally, an indirect way to treat HIV is based on using T-lymphocyte genome editing in order to render these lymphocytes resistant to HIV infection. The C–C chemokine receptor type 5 (CCR5) plays a major role as a co-receptor in the infection process. A naturally occurring CCR5-inactivating mutation, which is present in the European population, offers protection against AIDS in homozygous individuals. Gene editing tools to knock-out CCR5 in the genome of autologous cells using targeted CRISPR/Cas9 are thus being actively investigated. Several reports have described CRISPR/Cas9 mediated CCR5 ablation in cells such as hematopoietic stem cells (HSCs), which confers HIV-1 resistance *in vivo*.

## Bibliography

Anzalone AV, Randolph PB, Davis JR, Sousa AA, Koblan LW, Levy JM, Chen PJ, Wilson C, *et al*. Search-and-replace genome editing without double-strand breaks or donor DNA. *Nature*. 2019 Dec;576(7785):149–57. doi: 10.1038/s41586-019-1711-4.

Aubert M, Haick AK, Strongin DE, Klouser LM, Loprieno MA, Stensland L, Santo TK, Huang ML, Hyrien O, Stone D, Jerome KR. Gene editing for latent herpes simplex virus infection reduces viral load and shedding *in vivo*. *Nat Commun*. 2024 May 13;15(1):4018. doi: 10.1038/s41467-024-47940-y.

Chen L, Hong M, Luan C, Gao H, Ru G, Guo X, Zhang D, Zhang S, *et al.* Adenine transversion editors enable precise, efficient A•T-to-C•G base editing in mammalian cells and embryos. *Nat Biotechnol.* 2024 Apr;42(4): 638–50. doi: 10.1038/s41587-023-01821-9.

Chiesa R, Georgiadis C, Syed F, Zhan H, Etuk A, Gkazi SA, Preece R, Ottaviano G, *et al.* Base-edited CAR7 T cells for relapsed T-cell acute lymphoblastic leukemia. *N Engl J Med.* 2023 Sep 7;389(10):899–910. doi: 10.1056/ NEJMoa2300709.

Cowan QT, Komor AC. Genome editing with DNA-dependent polymerases. *Nat Biotechnol.* 2024 Aug 23. doi: 10.1038/s41587-024-02372-3.

Davis JR, Banskota S, Levy JM, Newby GA, Wang X, Anzalone AV, Nelson AT, Chen PJ, *et al.* Efficient prime editing in mouse brain, liver and heart with dual AAVs. *Nat Biotechnol.* 2024 Feb;42(2):253–64. doi: 10.1038/ s41587-023-01758-z.

Doman JL, Raguram A, Newby GA, Liu DR. Evaluation and minimization of Cas9-independent off-target DNA editing by cytosine base editors. *Nat Biotechnol.* 2020 May;38(5):620–8. doi: 10.1038/s41587-020-0414-6.

Ferrari S, Valeri E, Conti A, Scala S, Aprile A, Di Micco R, Kajaste-Rudnitski A, Montini E, Ferrari G, Aiuti A, Naldini L. Genetic engineering meets hematopoietic stem cell biology for next-generation gene therapy. *Cell Stem Cell.* 2023 May 4;30(5):549–70. doi: 10.1016/j.stem.2023.04.014.

Gaudelli NM, Komor AC, Rees HA, Packer MS, Badran AH, Bryson DI, Liu DR. Programmable base editing of A•T to G•C in genomic DNA without DNA cleavage. *Nature.* 2017 Nov 23;551(7681):464–71. doi: 10.1038/nature24644.

Ioannou A, Fontana M, Gillmore JD. RNA targeting and gene editing strategies for transthyretin amyloidosis. *BioDrugs.* 2023 Mar;37(2):127–42. doi: 10.1007/s40259-023-00577-7.

Jinek M, Chylinski K, Fonfara I, Hauer M, Doudna JA, Charpentier E. A programmable dual-RNA-guided DNA endonuclease in adaptive bacterial immunity. *Science.* 2012 Aug 17;337(6096):816–21. doi: 10.1126/science. 1225829.

Karpinski J, Hauber I, Chemnitz J, Schäfer C, Paszkowski-Rogacz M, Chakraborty D, Beschorner N, Hofmann-Sieber H, *et al.* Directed evolution of a recombinase that excises the provirus of most HIV-1 primary isolates with high specificity. *Nat Biotechnol.* 2016 Apr;34(4):401–9. doi: 10.1038/nbt.3467.

Khamaikawin W, Saisawang C, Tassaneetrithep B, Bhukhai K, Phanthong P, Borwornpinyo S, Phuphuakrat A, Pasomsub E, *et al*. CRISPR/Cas9 genome editing of CCR5 combined with C46 HIV-1 fusion inhibitor for cellular resistant to R5 and X4 tropic HIV-1. *Sci Rep*. 2024 May 13;14(1):10852. doi: 10.1038/s41598-024-61626-x.

Komor AC, Gaudelli NM. CRISPR-derived genome editing therapies: Progress from bench to bedside. *Mol Ther*. 2021 Nov 3;29(11):3125–39. doi: 10.1016/j.ymthe.2021.09.027.

Liu B, Dong X, Zheng C, Keener D, Chen Z, Cheng H, Watts JK, Xue W, Sontheimer EJ. Targeted genome editing with a DNA-dependent DNA polymerase and exogenous DNA-containing templates. *Nat Biotechnol*. 2024 Jul;42(7):1039–45. doi: 10.1038/s41587-023-01947-w.

Ngo W, Peukes JT, Baldwin A, Xue ZW, Hwang S, Stickels RR, Lin Z, Satpathy AT, Wells JA, Schekman R, Nogales E, Doudna JA. Mechanism-guided engineering of a minimal biological particle for genome editing. *bioRxiv*. 2024 Jul 24:2024.07.23.604809. doi: 10.1101/2024.07.23.604809.

Tong H, Wang X, Liu Y, Liu N, Li Y, Luo J, Ma Q, Wu D, *et al*. Programmable A-to-Y base editing by fusing an adenine base editor with an N-methylpurine DNA glycosylase. *Nat Biotechnol*. 2023 Aug;41(8):1080–4. doi: 10.1038/s41587-022-01595-6.

Torella L, Santana-Gonzalez N, Zabaleta N, Gonzalez Aseguinolaza G. Gene editing in liver diseases. *FEBS Lett*. 2024 Jul 30. doi: 10.1002/1873-3468.14989.

Wang Y, Liu M, Lin X, Wang H, Dong N, Liu H, Shao H, Zhang W. Genome editing of mammalian cells through RNA transcript-mediated homologous recombination repair. *Hum Gene Ther*. 2024 Aug;35(15-16):555–63. doi: 10.1089/hum.2024.025.

# Part II

# Genetic Pharmacology by Synthetic Oligonucleotides

# Chapter 10

# Antisense Deoxynucleotides

## 10.1 Introductory Remarks

In the beginning of the 20th century, Paul Ehrlich and Emil Fischer introduced the concepts of chemotherapy, magic bullet, and lock-key, in which a drug is defined as a small molecule which specifically binds to a biological target through a three-dimension spatial recognition pattern. With the advancement of genetics and the sequencing of the human genome, genetic defects, which are the cause of rare genetic diseases, cancer, and other conditions, are increasingly being elucidated. This has led to the emergence of a new class of "genetic" drugs. In addition to binding to their target through three-dimensional (3D) hydrogen bonding recognition pattern, these drugs recognize a one-dimension (1D) linear genetic sequence in their target DNA or RNA. In such cases, drug design is based on genetic information, which opens the perspective for the rapid and rational development of drugs against a considerable number of diseases characterized by specific genetic defects.

Theoretically, any gene or mRNA can be targeted by a nucleotide sequence selected to be unique within a given genome or transcriptome. Thus, such a sequence recognition mechanism opens tremendous possibilities in medicinal chemistry. Instead of painstaking and arduous customized search for specific 3D spatial recognition of a targeted biological ligand by a chemical compound or a monoclonal antibody, genetic drugs are based on a robust universal platform that can be used for a very large number of applications. Protein targets which were until now considered "non-druggable" can be challenged at the transcription and, more easily, at the translation level by targeting their corresponding mRNA. In addition, the use of a common validated technology for all antisense oligonucleotides (ASOs) or small interfering RNA (siRNA) allows shortening pharmaceutical development steps and reducing costs, which is of paramount importance for rare diseases. In the case of ultrarare diseases, personalized therapy can now be envisioned on these revolutionary platforms for as few as one single patient.

The basic concepts, principles, mechanisms of action, and chemical optimizations of ASOs and siRNAs are illustrated in Chapters 10 and 11. These RNA-targeting drugs can either lead to RNA degradation or act as steric blockers. In the latter case, they can inhibit RNA translation, antagonize a miRNA, modulate splicing, or induce exon skipping. To their specific, divergent functions correspond both specific chemical and delivery optimizations. Thus, RNA drugs can either restore therapeutic mRNA or, in most cases, suppress a pathologic mRNA or block mRNA translation to correct a "gain-of-function" dominant negative genetic disorder. Another important application is that of splice modulators or splice correctors, which can overcome a nonsense mutation and lead to the expression of a functional, albeit shortened, therapeutic protein.

## 10.2  Steric Blocker Antisense ASOs

The first ASO drug was introduced in 1978 against Rous sarcoma viral replication. It is a 13-mer synthetic oligodeoxynucleotide complementary to the 13 nucleotides of both the 3'- and 5'-reiterated terminal sequences of Rous sarcoma virus 35S RNA, to which the drug is annealing through Watson–Crick recognition. This creates an intracellular DNA-RNA heteroduplex, which may either function as a translational steric blocker or lead to mRNA degradation. The ASOs acting as steric blockers of translation target the mRNA translation initiation site (start codon). This inhibits, through steric hindrance, the binding of ribosomal subunits to the mRNA, thus blocking protein synthesis (Figure 10.1(A)).

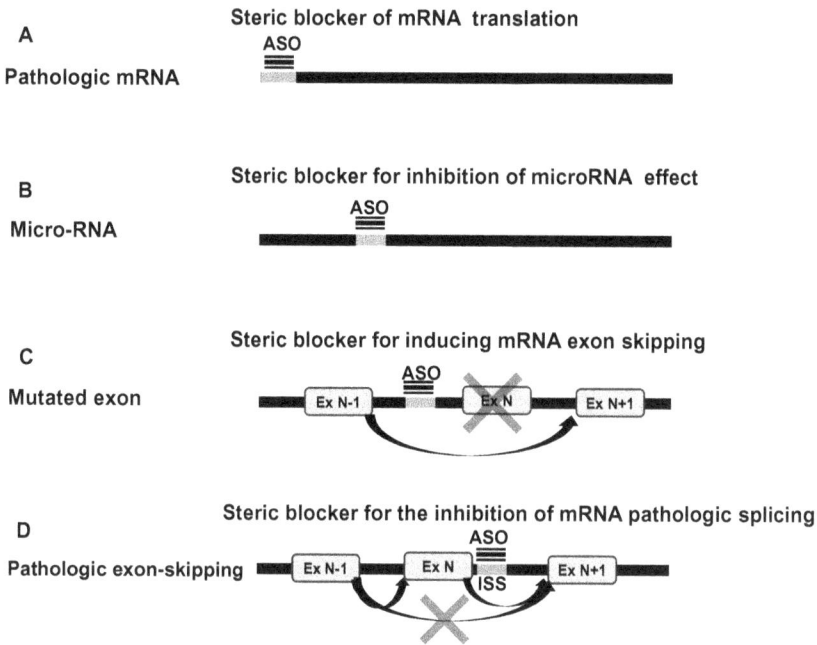

**Figure 10.1.** ASO steric blocking effects. In gray, the complementary targeted sequence on the mRNA is indicated. ISS: Intronic splice silencer. (A) mRNA Translation inhibition. (B) Antagomir. (C) ASO Inducing skipping of a pathologic exon which carries stop or out-of-frame mutations. (D) Splice corrector or splice modulator inhibits a non-desired naturally occurring exon skipping.

In addition to translation blockade, ASOs have the potential to exhibit various steric blocking effects, leading to significant therapeutic successes. These are schematized in Figure 10.1.

MicroRNAs (miRNAs) are a group of one to two thousand small non-coding RNA molecules which are made of 21–23 nucleotides. They play important biological functions as post-transcriptional regulators of gene expression. The miRNAs anneal to complementary sequences on mRNA molecules, leading to gene silencing by several mechanisms: mRNA cleavage mediated by the RNA-induced silencing complex RISC (see Chapter 11), mRNA destabilization by poly(A) tail shortening, or blocking of mRNA translation. As shown in Figure 10.1(B), ASO steric blocking can antagonize these cellular "bandmasters" and thus display an antagomir action, which presents interesting therapeutic applications in a large number of diseases.

An antisense blocker ASO can be used to sterically hinder a splice acceptor or splice enhancer site, thus promoting exon skipping (Figure 10.1(C)). This mechanism of action is of great interest for treating genetic diseases which are caused by stop or out-of-frame missense variants and where the skipping of one or of several exons leads to a still functional, or partially functional, truncated form of the protein product. This strategy has led to clinically approved ASO RNA drugs for Duchenne dystrophy. Exon skipping may also hold interest in cases where pathologic alternative splicing of variant genes occurs, which leads to the inclusion of an additional exon, thereby causing the expression of a nonfunctional protein. Finally, blocker ASOs can also treat cases where an intronic pathogenic variant results in aberrant inclusion of an intron segment into mRNA transcripts, thus abolishing protein function.

Figure 10.1(D) illustrates the use of an ASO to inhibit a naturally occurring undesired splicing event leading to exon N skipping and translation of a non-functional truncated protein. By blocking this undesired exon skipping, therapeutic restoration of a complete, functional protein is obtained. As will be described in Section 10.7, this splice correction is used in the case of spinal muscular atrophy (SMA), where a non-functional truncated form of the SMN2 mRNA is produced. An ASO which sterically blocks the intronic splice silencer present on the SMN2 gene favors pre-mRNA maturation toward a complete form of the SMN2 mRNA, thus leading to expression of a functional SMN protein. This approach has represented a historically major success as the first therapy for SMA. Another application of splice-corrector ASO is *sepofarsen*, which is an ASO designed to correct the splicing of the CEP290 gene for treating Leber congenital amaurosis 10 (LCA10), still in clinical development. Another application in clinical development is QR-421a, an antisense oligonucleotide designed to skip exon 13 of the USH2A gene. This approach aims to treat Usher syndrome type 2A and non-syndromic retinitis pigmentosa by restoring the production of functional usherin protein.

## 10.3 ASO-Induced mRNA Degradation by RNase H

While the antisense-mediated blockade of mRNA translation might be responsible for part of the observed decreased protein expression, it was later found that the loss of protein expression induced by ASOs was also due to mRNA degradation by ribonuclease H (RNase H). This RNase specifically recognizes RNA-DNA heteroduplexes and cleaves the associated mRNA. This nucleolytic mechanism of action drives most of the actual clinical applications of ASOs.

Eukaryotic cells are ubiquitously equipped with the enzyme ribonuclease H type 1 (designated here for simplicity as RNase H, instead of RNase H1) whose function is to remove RNA moieties from DNA and which plays a crucial role in the following cellular processes: (1) RNA primers are required to initiate the synthesis of both the leading strand and Okazaki fragments on the lagging DNA strand during genome replication; RNase H is responsible for removing these RNA primers from Okazaki fragments, which allows for the completion and joining of the DNA fragments. (2) DNA replicases occasionally incorporate ribonucleotides into DNA, and RNase H hydrolyzes the RNA strand in RNA–DNA hybrids, which is essential for maintaining genomic stability. (3) In retroviruses, RNase H activity is part of the reverse transcriptase enzyme, which helps degrade the RNA template after it has been copied into DNA. (4) Finally, R-loops are generated as a by-product of transcription when nascent mRNA molecules hybridize with the template DNA, which represents another example of naturally occurring RNA–DNA duplexes; RNase H helps in processing these three-stranded nucleic acid R-loop structures. Defects in RNase H can lead to severe consequences, such as embryo lethality in mice and Aicardi–Goutières syndrome in humans.

The RNase H nuclease belongs to the nucleotidyl-transferase superfamily, which relies on divalent cations to catalyze nucleophilic substitution reactions. These enzymatic reactions specifically hydrolyze either a single ribonucleotide or stretches of RNA in a diverse range of nucleic acids, such as RNA-DNA hybrids, R-loops, and double-stranded DNA with an embedded single ribonucleotide. Other enzymes such as transposase, retroviral integrase, Holliday junction resolvase, and RISC nuclease argonaute involved in the mechanism of RNA silencing belong to the same nucleotidyl-transferase superfamily as RNase H.

As shown in Figure 10.2, an ASO annealing to a complementary mRNA sequence creates an intracellular DNA–RNA heteroduplex to which RNase H binds, leading to cleavage and subsequent degradation of the targeted mRNA. After mRNA cleavage at the complementary site, the mRNA strand is released from the ASO, which thus becomes available for further association with another target mRNA.

RNase H-dependent ASOs are of interest for treating diseases caused by dominant-negative genetic variants. An important feature is that RNase H requires a non-modified deoxyribose moiety in the middle of the complementary ASO sequence (the "seed" sequence) to maintain its catalytic efficiency. Thus, an efficient ASO must be either a pure deoxy oligomer bearing only unmodified ribose sugars, or a gapmer, which contains a

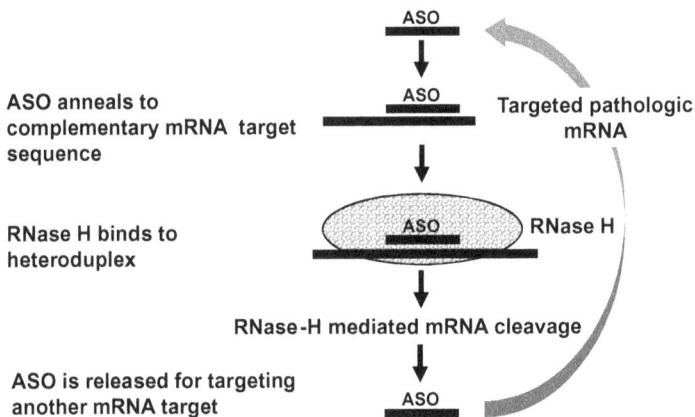

**Figure 10.2.** ASO-mediated mRNA degradation through RNase H nucleolytic activity. ASO (black rod) binds to a complementary sequence on mRNA. This heteroduplex induces RNase H binding and leads to mRNA cleavage. After mRNA cleavage, the mRNA fragments, ASO and RNase H, are released from each other. Gray arrow: Free ASO is recycled for binding to another mRNA on the target sequence, which induces a new cycle of RNase H binding and mRNA cleavage.

stretch of about 10 natural ribose sugars with a variable number of modified sugars on the 3' and 5' ends (see the following section).

## 10.4  ASO Chemical Optimization

After their initial discovery, the first enthusiastic attempts at the clinical use of both ASOs and siRNAs were very disappointing, leading to a drastic decrease in investment in these genetic pharmacology RNA drugs. These initial approaches used natural oligonucleotides, which have poor pharmacokinetics because they undergo rapid degradation by endo- and exonucleases. They degrade within 20 minutes after IV administration. In addition, these first generation ASOs and siRNAs were rapidly eliminated by kidney filtration, which decreases tissue distribution and might eventually induce undesirable toxicity to renal glomerules. Moreover, natural oligonucleotides are small, hydrophilic, polyanionic compounds due to the phosphodiester linkages, which hinder cell penetration through the lipophilic plasma membrane. Finally, the innate immune response to double-stranded RNA, particularly through the TLR3 receptor, was found to represent a strong bottleneck for the development of siRNA drugs (see Chapter 11). All these considerations led to the conclusion that chemical modifications were required for the ultimate success of the ASO or siRNA drug strategy.

Many comprehensive, reviews have been dedicated to the intensive chemistry efforts performed on ASO or siRNA derivatives, concerning their different components: backbone, sugar, and base. The most successful chemical modifications introduced to date on ASO and siRNA nucleotides are displayed in Figure 10.3. Because of their differing properties and modes of action, various chemical modifications have been selected over more than 20 years of intensive research for each class of RNA drugs.

The single-stranded nature of ASOs requires full phosphodiester backbone modification because of their high exposure to exo- and endonucleases. Figure 10.3(B) displays the most successful modified backbone linkage used to date, phosphorothioate (PS), in which a sulfur atom

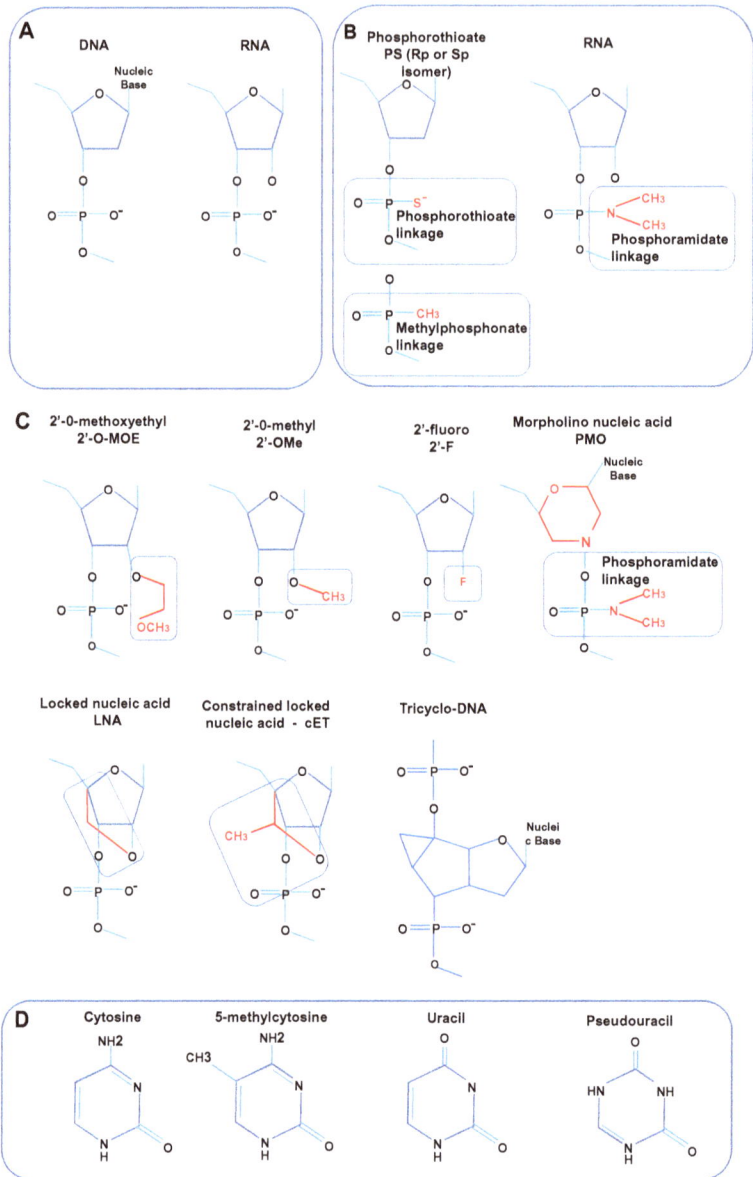

**Figure 10.3.**    Most popular nucleotide analogs used in ASO and siRNA drugs. (A) natural DNA (R=H) and RNA (R=OH) units; (B) linkage analog; (C) ribose analog; (D) base analog. 5-methyl cytosine is the only one that is currently being used in clinically approved drugs. Uracil and pseudouracil bases are also represented here because pseudouridine (Psi) is used in mRNA vaccines and mRNA drugs in place of uridine since it suppresses the detrimental innate immune response against double-stranded RNA stretches.

replaces one phosphate non-linking oxygen and which partially protects against nucleolytic activity. In addition, phosphorothioate modification has been shown to increase pharmacokinetics and cellular uptake. Indeed, the first ASO drug introduced to the market was the 21 nt full phosphorothioate oligodeoxynucleotide *fomivirsen* (Vitravene), which has the sequence 5'-GCG TTT GCT CTT CTT CTT GCG-3', targeting the CMV protein IE2 mRNA. Several other phosphodiester linkage modifications also confer nuclease resistance, for instance, methylphosphonate and phosphoramidate (Figure 10.3(B)), and mesylphosphoramidate, in which a methanesulfonyl (mesyl) group is attached to the phosphoramidate backbone.

It should be noted that each PS substitution introduces a chiral phosphate with two stereoisomers, the Sp and Rp forms. The Sp diastereoisomers are more resistant to nucleases and should be preferred for a blocking ASO. On the other hand, Rp diastereoisomers display a higher binding affinity and induce more efficient RNase H cleavage, which is more favorable for an mRNA degradation strategy. It has been shown that precise localization of Rp and Sp PS links could optimize the desired function and increase selectivity by decreasing off-target mismatch binding.

While phosphorothioate links confer improved relative nuclease resistance and metabolic stability, the protection is not complete. Moreover, PS links decrease ASO and siRNA binding affinity to the complementary mRNA. This can be corrected by introducing modifications into the ribose moiety. Modifications on the 2' carbon, such as 2'-fluoro, 2'-O-methyl, or 2'-O-metoxyethyl, are extensively used for both ASOs and siRNAs (Figure 10.3(C)). Another way to increase nuclease resistance is by introducing constraints in the ribose ring, such as in the bicyclic locked nucleic acids (LNAs) or in the constrained ethyl locked nucleic acids (cet-LNAs).

Other original structures, which are further modified from natural ribose or deoxyribose rings, have demonstrated their value in increasing metabolic stability while maintaining high binding affinity for mRNA. These are the morpholino, tricyclo-DNA, or PNA analogs (Figure 10.3(C)). Morpholino nucleic acids (commonly designated as PMOs) are methylene-morpholine rings linked through phosphorodiamidate groups instead of phosphates. They display a strong affinity for mRNA, leading to an efficient steric blocking effect. Preclinical and clinical studies have shown that PMOs demonstrate improved efficacy, excellent kinetic behavior, biological stability, and a good safety profile. Tricyclo-DNA oligomers display strong antisense and exon-skipping activities. PNAs are peptide nucleic acids in which the ribose-phosphodiester backbone has been replaced by the peptide linkage analog N-(2-aminoethyl)-glycine units, which allows the use of a convenient peptide synthesis technology. It has been reported, however, that PNAs have the disadvantage of rapid renal elimination.

Finally, base modifications have been introduced, such as the base analog 5-methylcytosine, because they increase nuclease resistance and reduce the innate immune response (Figure 10.3(D)). However, the risk of genomic incorporation of these non-natural bases has hindered their clinical use so far, except for 5-methyl cytosine. In addition, pseudouridine (Psi) displayed in Figure 10.3(D) is not used in anti-RNA nucleotidic drugs; rather, it is used in the composition of mRNA vaccines to alleviate the innate immune response against double-stranded RNA stretches.

More chemical refinements have been proposed to improve the pharmacokinetics and blocking properties of ASOs. For instance, it was found that a mixture of LNA with 2'-O-methyl and 2'F nucleotide, together with a PS backbone, was most efficient at inhibiting miRNAs. Such mixed oligomers are called "mixmers" and are schematized in Figure 10.4.

Other means to improve ASO bioavailability at the desired tissues and cells include nanoparticle encapsulation (see Chapter 6 on the chemical delivery of non-viral vectors) and covalent coupling to a penetration enhancer or targeting moiety. Coupling morpholino nucleic acids to a peptide rich in alanine and the cationic amino-acid arginine has been reported to increase tissue delivery and the efficacy of exon skipping or exon restoration in models of Duchenne dystrophy and spinal muscular atrophy. Linking ASO to a fatty acid chain showed promising results in a spinal muscular atrophy model. The use of triantennary N-acetyl-galactosamine (GalNac) for targeting and high-performance delivery to liver hepatocytes via the asialoglycoprotein receptor represents one of the most successful strategies both for ASOs and siRNAs (see Section 6.8 of Chapter 6).

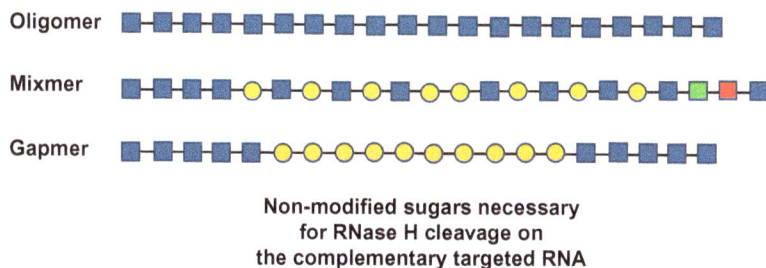

Non-modified sugars necessary
for RNase H cleavage on
the complementary targeted RNA

**Figure 10.4.** Diverse types of ASOs developed at the preclinical and clinical stages. Squares, circles, and assorted colors represent the diverse types of nucleotides displayed in Figure 10.3. The linkage between each nucleotide might also vary, for instance the phosphorothioate Sp and Rp diastereoisomers. In a gapmer, the yellow circles represent non-modified nucleotides allowing cleavage by RNase H of the annealed, complementary mRNA.

This technology has led to impressive therapeutic achievements. Attempts to deliver ASOs through the intestine and blood–brain barrier have been reported, with results still to be confirmed however.

Enhanced bioavailability and nuclease resistance are sufficient conditions for achieving the distinct therapeutic mechanisms of action of ASOs, as illustrated in Figure 10.1: steric block of mRNA translation, microRNA inhibition (antagomir effect), exon skipping, and exon restoration. Several Food and Drug Administration (FDA)-approved drugs demonstrate the success of these chemical modifications in treating rare diseases, which will be further detailed in the following by taking principally muscular and neuronal diseases as a selection of illustrative examples. However, it has to be noted that the field of potential applications is much larger, covering brain degenerative disorders such as Huntington's chorea, other triplet expansion diseases, cancers, infectious diseases, hypercholesterolemia, and liver metabolic disorders.

## 10.5 ASO Chemical Optimization for RNase H-Induced mRNA Cleavage

The necessity to maintain RNase H activity represents a major constraint which limits the use of many of the chemical modifications presented above. The phosphorothioate linkage is compatible with RNase H activity. Inversely, methylphosphonate substitution must be finely optimized. In a typical model study, heteroduplexes formed with natural deoxyoligonucleotides or phosphorothioate analogs led to mRNA cleavage by RNase H, whereas a duplex formed with an oligonucleotide containing six methylphosphonate deoxynucleosides alternating with normal deoxynucleotides was not permissive to RNase H attack. The mRNA's susceptibility to cleavage by RNase H increased in parallel to a reduction in the number of methylphosphonate linkages.

Sugar modifications such as morpholino or LNA are not tolerated by RNase H. Uniformly modified 2'-deoxy-2'-fluoro phosphorothioate oligonucleotides lead to antisense molecules with strong binding affinity, high selectivity for the RNA target, and stability toward nucleases; however, they do not support RNase H nucleolytic activity on mRNA. Conversely, incorporating a mixture of these modifications into "chimeric" oligonucleotides has been shown to activate mammalian RNase H-mediated degradation. Consequently, a sizable proportion of RNase H-dependent ASOs are "gapmers," in which a gap of 10 unmodified deoxyribose is flanked by 3' and 5' "wings" whose partial composition in chemically modified nucleotides leads to metabolic stability, enhanced binding to the target, and cellular availability (Figure 10.4).

A large variety of gapmer geometries can be envisioned. A reduced gap size confers more precision in the cleavage zone and potentially contributes to allele specificity. Different flanking wings have been proposed with the aim of increasing affinity and selectivity for the target RNA. However, care should be taken to ensure that the cleaved mRNA dissociates to initiate another mRNA degradation. Thus, ASO affinity for the mRNA target must not be too high. For instance, with LNA-containing wings, an increased binding affinity has been reported, which leads to an optimal size of 12–15 nucleotides. In contrast, gapmer *inotersen* (Tegsedi), which is clinically approved for treating transthyretin amyloidosis, is a fully phosphorothioate modified ASO with five 2'-O-methoxyethyl ribonucleotides on each side, thus consisting of a 5-10-5 structure. In addition, a too strong affinity might induce off-target binding and RNase H cleavage of mismatched mRNAs. Because a high ASO concentration is observed in the liver, off-target hepatic toxicity has been reported for 2'fluoro and LNAs.

## 10.6  Exon-Skipping ASO for Duchenne Muscular Dystrophy

Duchenne muscular dystrophy (DMD) is caused by anomalies in the dystrophin gene located on the X chromosome (Xp21.2). Because the dystrophin gene is the largest one in human genomes, genetic variants and deletions occur at a higher frequency than those of other genes, and DMD has one of the highest prevalence among rare diseases (about 6 in 100,000). Diagnosis is suspected based on the clinical picture, family history, and laboratory findings (serum creatine kinase being 100–200 times the normal level). Genetic testing is a critical tool for accurate DMD diagnosis (Orphanet code 98896).

DMD onset occurs in early childhood, and affected boys may exhibit a delay in walking accompanied with speech and/or global developmental impairments. Autism and behavioral issues, such as attention deficit hyperactivity disorder (ADHD), anxiety, and obsessive-compulsive disorder are observed. Untreated DMD children rarely achieve the ability to run or jump. The condition progresses rapidly; as a result, the child develops a waddling gait and exhibits a positive Gowers' sign. Proximal muscles are affected first, followed by distal limb muscle. Climbing stairs becomes difficult, and the child falls frequently. Loss of independent ambulation occurs between the ages of 6 and 13 years, with an average of 9.5 years among non-steroid-treated patients. Once ambulation is lost, joint contractures and scoliosis develop rapidly. Until recently, untreated patients might not survive beyond late teens to early twenties because of respiratory failure and/or cardiomyopathy; however, life expectancy is now increasing thanks to adapted cardiac care and assisted ventilation.

DMD belongs to the larger group of rare genetic progressive muscular dystrophies called dystrophinopathies, which also include Becker muscular dystrophy (BMD) and a symptomatic form in female carriers. Dystrophinopathies present a spectrum of severity, ranging from progressive skeletal and cardiac muscle wasting and weakness (DMD and BMD) to less severe muscle weakness or isolated cardiomyopathy affecting carrier females. At the mildest end of the spectrum, exercise-induced muscle cramps and myoglobinuria may be the only features, while at the most severe end, there may be a complete loss of muscle function, cardiomyopathy, and respiratory failure. BMD presents a mild phenotype and a broad spectrum of clinical severity, with onset of symptoms occurring from early childhood to as late as age 60. A very severe, rapidly progressive, X-linked dilated cardiomyopathy (Orphanet code 262) may also be caused by mutations in the dystrophin gene.

Muscle damage in DMD is caused by the complete absence of the cytoplasmic sarcolemmal protein dystrophin, which participates in a complex connecting the muscle fiber cytoskeleton to the surrounding extracellular matrix through the cell membrane. Dystrophin protects myotube integrity during muscle contraction. Dystrophin possesses a central rod domain of 24 spectrin-like repeats. Its primary muscular transcript measures about 2,100 kilobases. The mature mRNA, which is formed by the junction of 79 exons, measures 14.0 kilobases and encodes a protein consisting of 3,685 amino acid residues. Hence, intensive splicing is necessary for dystrophin biosynthesis.

Dystrophinopathies are allelic conditions caused by deletions, duplications, and mutations in the dystrophin gene. While DMD genetic variants are frameshifted, BMD variants are in-frame. While severe DMD results from complete absence of dystrophin, the moderate BMD form is only observed when one or several of the spectrin-like repeats are missing. Deletions identified in DMD patients shift the translational open reading frame (ORF), thus resulting in an incomplete, abnormal protein product of which the COOH terminal fragment may be non-functional or lost. In contrast, in BMD patient deletions maintain in frame the translational ORF for amino acids and predict a shorter protein with lower molecular weight. This indicates that the smaller protein product, devoid of a certain number of internal spectrin-like domains, remains semi-functional, resulting in the milder Becker clinical phenotype. From this observation, it was predicted that, for some DMD patients, an in-frame skipping of the exon containing a nonsense mutation or deletion could have therapeutic value. Figure 10.5 illustrates an exon skipping obtained through the binding of a steric blocker ASO targeting an intronic splice acceptor, donor site, or exonic splice enhancer site.

Given the fact that several thousand variants have been reported among DMD patients, a search identified which in-frame exon skipping proved favorable for treating a high proportion of them. As shown in Figure 10.6, skipping exon 51 results in an in-frame skipping and leads to a partially functional protein in several deletion scenarios. Other partially internally shortened proteins would contain the following junctional exons: 50–53, 49–52, 49–52, 48–52, 47–52, 46–52, and 44–52. The deletions displayed in Figure 10.6 correspond to about 15–17% of the DMD population.

An elegant *in vivo* exon skipping proof of concept leading to the expression of a partially functional dystrophin molecule devoid of a certain

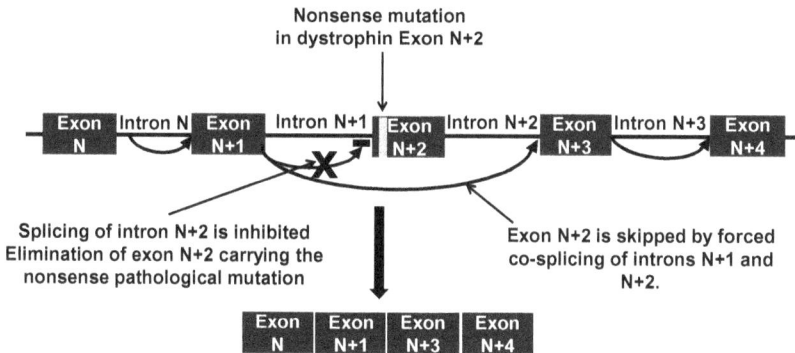

**Figure 10.5.**   Therapeutic exon skipping. An ASO targeting and blocking an intronic splice acceptor, donor site, or exonic splice enhancer site enforces exon skipping. In the case of the picture, the ASO targets, binds to, and sterically blocks the acceptor site of intron N+1, resulting in the skipping of exon N+2. The exons N+1 and N+3 must be in frame to ensure the expression of a protein devoid of only exon N+2, which may still be fully or partially functional.

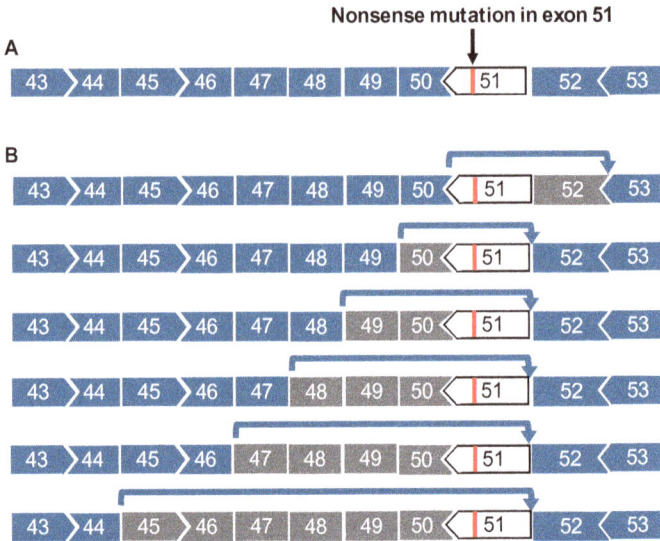

**Figure 10.6.** (A) Exons 43–53 of the integral dystrophin gene. (B) In gray, the group of exons whose concomitant in frame deletion could, in theory, lead to a shortened functional or semi-functional dystrophin protein comprising only the protein encoded by the exons in dark blue and allowing to skip the mutated exon 51.

number of spectrin-like domains was obtained by using an AAV viral vector delivering an antisense moiety borne by a U7 or U1 small nuclear RNA carrying a specific sequence, inducing exon 51 skipping in a mouse model. The muscle force recovery was restored in these experiments. These highly promising results prompted the development of synthetic steric blocker ASOs. This has led to the drug *eteplirsen* (AVI-4658; Exondys 51), which has been approved by the FDA but not by the European Medicine Agency (EMA), suggesting that its efficacy is a matter of debate. *Eteplirsen* is a 30 nucleotide morpholino nucleotide oligomer delivered intravenously. Its sequence is CTCCAACATCAAGGAAGATGGCATTTCTAG.

Other commercialized ASOs for DMD induce the skipping of exons 53 and 45 (*golodirsen and casimersen*, respectively), and in 2024, there were four ASOs on the market for DMD, all being morpholinos. Other chemistries were in clinical development: 2'-MOE-PS 20-mer ASO and peptide-conjugated ASO.

## 10.7 Steric Splice Corrector ASO for Spinal Muscular Atrophy

Spinal muscular atrophy (SMA) is the second most common fatal disease of infants. It is a rare autosomal-recessive neuromuscular disease that affects 1 in 6,000 children and is characterized by progressive general muscle waste. SMA is caused by mutations or deletions in the Survival Motoneuron 1 gene (SMN1). The gene for SMA was mapped to chromosome 5q13 within the telomeric region. This 20 kb gene encodes a 294 amino acid protein.

SMA displays various levels of severity. The less severe forms are classified as Type II, Type III, and Type IV, based on the age of onset and ultimate motor disability. The most severe form is Type I (Werdnig–Hoffmann disease), which occurs in about 60% of cases and is associated with quadriplegia, respiratory muscle paralysis, and mortality shortly after birth. Werdnig–Hoffmann patients are never able to sit by themselves and require support for their nutrition and ventilatory functions. SMA patients who can sit but are unable to walk without assistance are classified as Type II. Milder Type III SMA patients possess sitting and walking abilities; however, they typically lose their ability to walk by adulthood. Type IV patients have a normal life expectancy but develop muscle weakness over time.

Homozygous deletions or deleterious mutations in the SMN1 gene are present in all SMA patients. The SMN2 gene is a paralog of SMN1 which results from the duplication of the 5q13 chromosomal region and has been identified to be located in a more centromeric position. The SMN2 gene is unique to *Homo sapiens* and differs from SMN1 by fewer than 20 nucleotides; however, its functional significance lies in the presence of a thymine rather than a cytosine in exon 7.

This difference between SMN1 and SMN2 genes is of crucial clinical importance because the cytosine replacement by thymine inactivates a splicing enhancer and, conversely, creates a splicing silencer in the pre-mRNA. Consequently, exon 7 is skipped by the splicing machinery in about 90% of matured SMN2 mRNA, leading to an unstable, non-functional, shorter SMN2 protein (Figure 10.7). Still, about 10% of

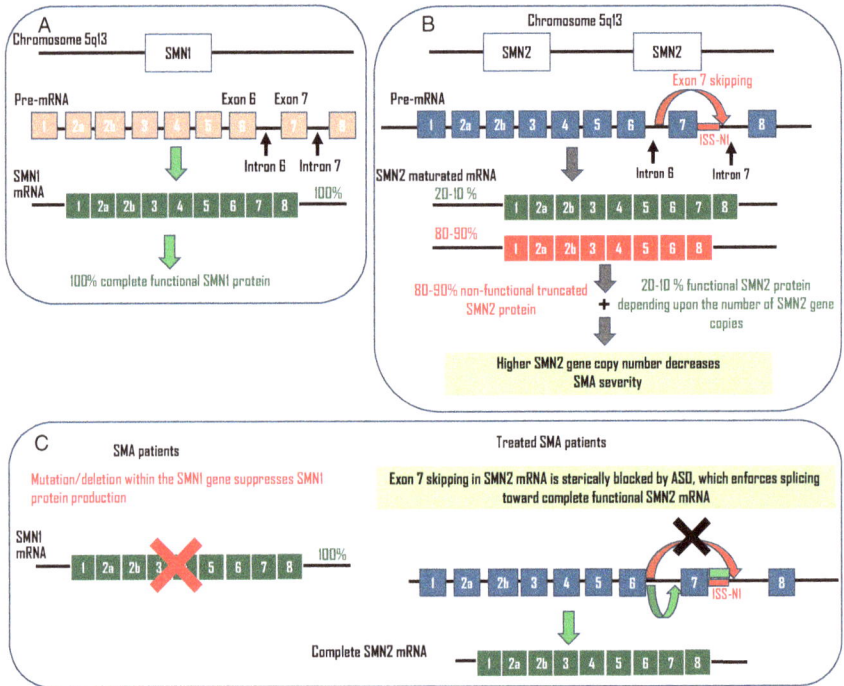

**Figure 10.7.** Summary of the genetic and molecular defects causing several levels of SMA severity and illustration of the treatment by a steric blocker ASO. (A) In non-affected individuals, both SMN1 and SMN2 genes are wild type. SMN1 pre-mRNA is transcribed and matured into complete mRNA, corresponding to the nine exons: 1, 2a, 2b, 3, 4, 5, 6, 7, and 8. This leads to the production of a fully functional SMN1 protein, a process which does not occur in SMA patients, who have a nonsense mutation or deletion of the SMN1 gene. (B) The SMN2 paralog gene contains several sequences which negatively impact the correct splicing and impair the incorporation of the exon 7 sequence into the mature SMN2 mRNA. The most important of these inhibitory sequences is the intronic splicing silencer N1 (ISS N1), located in 5' end of intron 7. Therefore, only a 10–20% minority of SMN2 transcripts contain all the necessary exonic sequences for a functional SMN2 protein. About 80–90% of SMN2 transcripts are translated into a shortened, non-functional SMN2 protein devoid of exon 7, which is unstable. The presence of multiple copies of the SMN2 gene results in a higher quantity of functional SMN2 being produced, and partially alleviates the disease severity. Type I patients generally possess two SMN2 gene copies; Type II have three SMN2 gene copies; and Types III and IV have four SMN2 gene copies. (C) In SMA patients, a mutation/deletion induces the loss of SMN1 protein production. A splice corrector ASO, designed as a steric blocker of ISS N1, very efficiently increases the level of complete fully competent SMN2 protein and has been clinically validated as the drug *nusinersen* (Spinraza).

mature SMN2 transcripts contain exon 7 and lead to a functional SMN2 protein with neuroprotective properties identical to those of SMN1.

The SMN2 gene is located in an unstable chromosomal region and is consequently present at varying copy numbers in the population, leading to variable production of functional SMN2 protein. The breadth of the severity spectrum of the SMA disease has been correlated with the number of SMN2 copies, which is coherent with the assumption that more SMN2 copies may, at least partially, compensate for the absence of SMN1 protein. As schematized in Figure 10.7, the presence of multiple copies of the SMN2 gene partially alleviates the disease symptoms by allowing more functional SMN2 protein to be produced, with Type I patients generally possessing two SMN2 copies, Type II having three SMN2 copies, and Type III having three or four SMN2 gene copies. Thus, the number of SMN2 copies is inversely correlated with SMA severity; however, other genes have also been proposed to influence its severity.

The observation that SMN2 is a strong disease modifier established the basis for the quest to increase the production of a complete and functional SMN2 protein by antagonizing the unwanted exon 7 skipping reaction. Through a systematic study of minigene mutants with different deletion at the 5' end of intron 7, a novel inhibitory element located immediately downstream of the 5' splice site in intron 7 was identified, which was called intronic splicing silencer N1 (ISS-N1). A pragmatic approach consisting of screening a large number of overlapping ASOs targeting introns 6 and 7, as well as exon 7, identified several sites on the three sequences, whose steric blocking would inhibit the undesired skipping of SMN2 exon 7, and confirmed that ISS-N1 was the most promising target sequence for enforcing full SMN2 protein expression. Thus, several ASOs targeting a sequence at approximately 10 nucleotides downstream of the 5' splice site were further developed, leading to the "splice corrector" drug *nusinersen* (Spinraza).

*Nusinersen* (Spinraza) was made available in 2016 as the first treatment for spinal amyotrophy. Remarkably, the *nusinersen* discovery rationale was based on the above-described thorough elucidation of the molecular mechanism of SMN1 and SMN2 mRNA maturation.

*Nusinersen* increases child survival and is administered via repeated intrathecal delivery (i.e., in the spinal cord). *Nusinersen* is an 18 nucleotide oligomer whose 5'-3' sequence is UCACUUUCAUAAUGCUGG. It is a highly modified ASO, possessing a full phosphorothioate backbone and 2'-O-MOE (2'-O-methoxyethyl)-modified ribose to increase metabolic resistance and bioavailability. In addition, all pyrimidines are 5-methylated: uracil replaced by thymine, and cytosine replaced by 5'-methyl cytidyl. The *nusinersen* IUPAC formula is detailed in Table 10.1.

**Table 10.1.**   *Nusinersen* and *inotersen* IUPAC formulas.

*Nusinersen* condensed IUPAC formula:
Thy-MeOEt(-2)Ribf-sP-m5Cyt-MeOEt(-2)Ribf-sP-Ade-MeOEt(-2)Ribf-sP-m5Cyt-
    MeOEt(-2)Ribf-sP-Thy-MeOEt(-2)Ribf-sP-Thy-MeOEt(-2)Ribf-sP-Thy-MeOEt(-2)
    Ribf-sP-m5Cyt-MeOEt(-2)Ribf-sP-Ade-MeOEt(-2)Ribf-sP-Thy-MeOEt(-2)Ribf-sP-
    Ade-MeOEt(-2)Ribf-sP-Ade-MeOEt(-2)Ribf-sP-Thy-MeOEt(-2)Ribf-sP-Gua-
    MeOEt(-2)Ribf-sP-m5Cyt-MeOEt(-2)Ribf-sP-Thy-MeOEt(-2)Ribf-sP-Gua-MeOEt(-2)
    Ribf-sP-Gua-MeOEt(-2)Ribf.

*Nusinersen* detailed IUPAC formula:
O2'-(2-methoxyethyl)-5-methyl-P-thio-uridylyl-(3'->5')-O2'-(2-methoxyethyl)-5-
    methyl-P-thio-cytidylyl-(3'->5')-O2'-(2-methoxyethyl)-P-thio-adenylyl-(3'->5')-O2'-
    (2-methoxyethyl)-5-methyl-P-thio-cytidylyl-(3'->5')-O2'-(2-methoxyethyl)-5-methyl-
    P-thio-uridylyl-(3'->5')-O2'-(2-methoxyethyl)-5-methyl-P-thio-uridylyl-(3'->5')-O2'-
    (2-methoxyethyl)-5-methyl-P-thio-uridylyl-(3'->5')-O2'-(2-methoxyethyl)-5-methyl-
    P-thio-cytidylyl-(3'->5')-O2'-(2-methoxyethyl)-P-thio-adenylyl-(3'->5')-O2'-(2-
    methoxyethyl)-5-methyl-P-thio-uridylyl-(3'->5')-O2'-(2-methoxyethyl)-P-thio-
    adenylyl-(3'->5')-O2'-(2-methoxyethyl)-P-thio-adenylyl-(3'->5')-O2'-(2-
    methoxyethyl)-5-methyl-P-thio-uridylyl-(3'->5')-O2'-(2-methoxyethyl)-P-thio-
    guanylyl-(3'->5')-O2'-(2-methoxyethyl)-5-methyl-P-thio-cytidylyl-(3'->5')-O2'-(2-
    methoxyethyl)-5-methyl-P-thio-uridylyl-(3'->5')-O2'-(2-methoxyethyl)-P-thio-
    guanylyl-(3'->5')-O2'-(2-methoxyethyl)-guanosine

*Inotersen* compacted IUPAC formula:
Thy-MeOEt(-2)Ribf-sP-m5Cyt-MeOEt(-2)Ribf-sP-Thy-MeOEt(-2)Ribf-sP-Thy-
    MeOEt(-2)Ribf-sP-Gua-MeOEt(-2)Ribf-sP-dGuo-sP-dThd-sP-dThd-sP-dAdo-sP-
    m5Cyt-dRibf-sP-dAdo-sP-dThd-sP-dGuo-sP-dAdo-sP-dAdo-sP-Ade-MeOEt(-2)
    Ribf-sP-Thy-MeOEt(-2)Ribf-sP-m5Cyt-MeOEt(-2)Ribf-sP-m5Cyt-MeOEt(-2)
    Ribf-sP-m5Cyt-MeOEt(-2)Ribf

As a splice corrector, *nusinersen* displays high efficacy in promoting exon 7 recovery into SMN2 protein. It was shown that increasing SMN exclusively in peripheral tissues completely rescued muscle necrosis in mild SMA mouse models and robustly extended survival in severe SMA mice, with significant improvements in vulnerable tissues and motor function. However, CNS effects upon IV injection could only be observed in neonates but not in adult mice. It is known that the blood–brain barrier is permeable in neonates and subsequently closes itself concomitantly with the expression of tight junctions and the Glut1 glucose transporter in capillary endothelium. This suggests that the PS- 2′O-Me ASOs *nusinersen* did not cross the blood–brain barrier. However, direct administration of *nusinersen* into the cerebrospinal fluid or the brain parenchyma allows for reasonable distribution through the brain and spinal cord, the latter being an absolute requirement for SMA.

Well-thought clinical development allowed to prove the clinical benefit of intrathecal splice corrector *nusinersen* for Type I SMA in only a few years. The results obtained from patients were so spectacular that FDA approval was obtained within about three months, which represents one of the shortest approval duration ever observed. Further Phase IV clinical data have shown that the earlier the treatment is given after birth, the better the clinical results. This opened the way to systematic SMA newborn genetic screening in various countries, which was not the case before. Multiple other candidate ASOs are being tested as SMN2 splice modifiers, such as an LNA/DNA mixmer. Remarkably, quite a short while after the revolutionary *nusinersen* commercialization, two other approaches led to approved drugs against SMA. *Onasemnogene abeparvovec* (Zolgensma) is a self-complementary AAV-9 vector capable of crossing the blood–brain barrier, carrying the SMN1 cDNA sequence, which has shown positive results with systemic IV administration and has been approved by the FDA and the EMA. *Risdiplam* (Evrysdi) is an orally administered splicing modifier of SMN2, which increases the level of functional SMN2 protein. *Risdiplam's* large domain of application covers all types of SMA, and it has been approved in the USA, Japan, and Europe as a treatment which does not necessitate hospital intervention.

## 10.8   RNase H-Dependent ASO *Inotersen* for Treating Hereditary Transthyretin Amyloidosis

Hereditary transthyretin amyloidosis (hATTR) is a rare, gain-of-function genetic disease. It represents a paramount example of clinical success for RNA drugs inducing mRNA degradation because both ASO and siRNA drugs have reached clinical use. This disease represents the first indication for a clinically approved siRNA. Moreover, two siRNA drugs with different delivery principles have been approved for hATTR within a brief period of time (see Chapter 11).

The transthyretin protein (TTR) is secreted by the liver, choroid plexus, and the retinal pigment epithelium. Its important function is to transport thyroid hormone thyroxine (T4) and retinol in the whole body. TTR is a 55 kDa homotetramer, which is formed by the initial association of dimers and subsequent dimer–dimer binding. hATTR is a group of several dominant-negative diseases related to variants in the TTR gene. More than 140 different TTR variants have been identified. In these rare hereditary diseases, mutant TTR misfolding leads to the formation of amyloid aggregates which accumulate in various tissues and cause various pathologies: hATTR, familial amyloid polyneuropathy (FAP), and familial amyloid cardiomyopathy (FAC). Cardiomyopathy results from myocardial infiltration of abnormal amyloid protein. In addition to polyneuropathy and cardiomyopathy, other transthyretin amyloidosis symptoms involve nephropathy and ocular pathology. Moreover, wild-type transthyretion amyloidosis (wtATTR) has been observed as being caused by normal wild-type transthyretin, which primarily occurs in older patients. So, any treatment developed for the small population affected by hereditary transthyretin amyloidosis might also prove useful for the very large population of individuals aged over 80 years.

Before the introduction of RNA drugs, hATTR treatment involved liver transplantation and, more recently, the small molecule drugs *diflunisal* and *tafamidis* (Vyndaqel, Vyndamax), which stabilize TTR in a non-aggregating form. Since recent years, however, an extremely efficient treatment to hATTR with polyneuropathy has been achieved through

RNA drugs that decrease liver TTR mRNA. Both RNases-H dependent ASOs, such as *inotersen* (Tegsedi), and RISC-dependent siRNA *patisiran* (Onpattro) and *vutrisiran* (Amvuttra) (Chapter 11) have successfully reached the market.

The ASO *inotersen* (Tegsedi) is a 20-mer gapmer similar to that depicted in Figure 10.4. It leads to the degradation of TTR mRNA, with minimal off-target effects. It is fully PS-modified (phosphorothioate backbone), with five ribose on both the 5' and 3' ends carrying 2'-O-methoxyethyl (2'-MOE) moieties. The 10 central nucleotides have a natural ribose. The nucleotide sequence of *inotersen* is UCUUGGTTACATGAAAUCCC, with the nucleotides UCUUG and AUCCC carrying a 2'-OMOE. As for *nusinersen*, all cytosines and uracil of *inotersen* are 5'-methylated (uracil replaced by thymine and cytosine by 5-methyl cytosine). The *inotersen* IUPAC formula is detailed in Table 10.1.

After subcutaneous (SC) injection, *inotersen* leads to a robust decreasing effect on the levels of both variant and wild-type transthyretin. It clearly inhibits TTR production and slows down the progression of the disease; however, it does not seem to induce any reverse effects on already-formed amyloid aggregates. Reported *inotersen* adverse events include thrombocytopenia. This could be linked to the presence of phosphorothioate linkages, which have been shown to be a potent platelet activator, as well as contributing to a risk of glomerulonephritis and hepatic toxicity.

## 10.9  RNase H-Dependent ASO for Treating Eye Disorders and Amyotrophic Lateral Sclerosis

As mentioned, the eye was the first organ in which ASOs entered clinical use. The first ASO which has been introduced is *fomivirsen* (brand name: Vitravene) for the treatment of cytomegalovirus (CMV) retinitis in AIDS patients. It was approved by the FDA in 1998. *Fomivirsen* works by targeting the CMV mRNA, thereby inhibiting the replication of the virus. It was specifically used for patients with CMV retinitis, who were intolerant of, or had contraindications to, other treatments.

Another eye indication in clinical development is QR-1123, an ASO targeting the P23H mutation in the rhodopsin (RHO) gene. It works by selectively knocking down the mutant mRNA, thereby reducing the production of the toxic protein associated with autosomal dominant retinitis pigmentosa.

Amyotrophic lateral sclerosis (ALS), also known as motor neuron disease (MND) or Lou Gehrig's disease, is a rare but terminal neurodegenerative disorder. It is caused by the progressive loss of both upper and lower motor neurons, which normally control voluntary muscle contraction. ALS is characterized by a progressive degeneration of motor neurons in the cerebral cortex, leading to the destruction of the pyramidal tract (involving the first motor neuron), and the neurons of the anterior horn of the spinal cord, leading to the destruction of associated motor units (involving the second motor neuron). This causes a progressive paralysis of the skeletal muscles in the limbs, trunk (including respiratory muscles), and the head. The disease often presents in its initial stages gradual muscle stiffness, twitches, and weakness, and motor neuron loss typically continues until the abilities to eat, speak, move, and finally breathe are all lost.

The causes of ALS are considered multifactorial, affecting both sexes, and its incidence increases with age starting at 40 years. In the USA and Canada, it is also named after Lou Gehrig, a renowned baseball player who died from the disease in 1941.

Very few treatments are available for ALS. Since the introduction in 1995 of the drug riluzole, which offers some increase in life expectancy, no progress had been described and many clinical rials had failed. This was until the drug *tofersen* (Qalsody) was approved for medical use in the United States in 2023. The FDA considered it to be a first-in-class medication. *Tofersen* is an ASO that targets the production of superoxide dismutase 1 (SOD1), an enzyme whose mutant form is associated with ALS in 15% of familial cases, which themselves represent 10–15% of total number of SLA cases. A mutation in the SOD1 gene is also observed in about 1% of sporadic cases. Thus, about 2% of all patients affected by ALS, a dreadful disease, can benefit from this ASO. *Tofersen* is

Antisense strand 5' to 3'

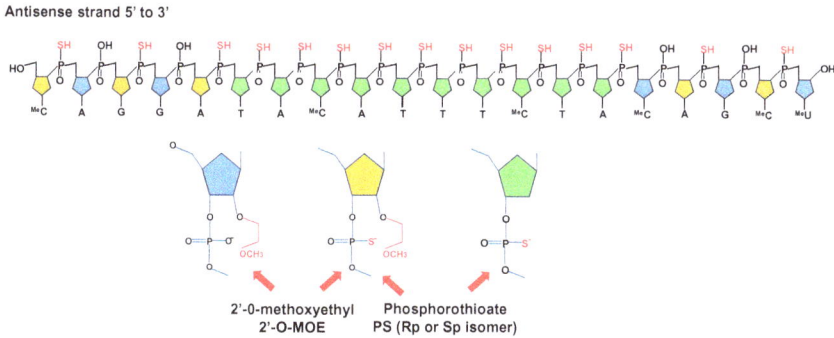

**Figure 10.8.** Tofersen formula.

administered as an intrathecal injection in order to obtain a therapeutic decrease in the mutated SOD1 protein production in the nervous system.

*Tofersen* is a 20-base residue (20-mer) 5-10-5 MOE gapmer mixed backbone ASO (Figure 10.8). Of the 19 internucleotide linkages, 15 are 3'-O to 5'-O phosphorothioate diesters, and four are 3'-O to 5'-O phosphate diesters. Ten of the 20 sugar residues are 2-deoxy-D-ribose, and the other ribose are modified by a 2'-O-(2-methoxyethyl) (MOE) group. The residues are arranged such that there are five MOE nucleosides at the 5' and 3' ends of the molecule, flanking a gap of 10 2'-deoxynucleosides. The cytosine and uridine bases are methylated at the 5' position. The molecular formula is C230 H317 N72 O123 P19 S15 and the molecular weight is 7127.86 atomic mass units.

## 10.10 Type 1 Myotonic Dystrophy: Different Proposed ASO Modes of Action

Myotonic dystrophy (or also called dystrophic myotonia) is a multisystemic disease with a frequency of 1 in 8,000 worldwide. The most severe form (DM1) includes symptoms such as myotonia, muscle weakness, cardiac arrhythmias, cognitive dysfunction, and cataracts. The genetic cause of DM1 stems from repeated expansion of a CTG triplet motif in the DM Protein Kinase (DMPK) gene. Normal DMPK gene contains 5–37 repeats, while a variant DM1 DMPK gene may contain up to thousands of CTG repeats, and the number of repeats correlates with disease severity.

Variant DMPK mRNAs form hairpin structures made from CUG repeats and assemble in well-characterized nuclear foci. The molecular mechanism of DM1 pathology results from the toxicity of these nuclear foci, which bind and sequester proteins of the muscleblind-like (MBNL) family, thus interfering with the MBNL proteins natural splicing functions. The mis-splicing reactions, due to insufficient availability of the MBNL protein in the nucleus, induce a fetal-like pattern in adult DM1 cells. This fetal-like character concerns a multiplicity of proteins, such as the muscle chlorine channel, insulin receptor, cardiac troponin T, bypass integrator 1, skeletal rapid troponin T, dystrophin (DMD), and cardiac sodium channel SCN5A. This general splicing defect, called spliceopathy, leads to myotonia and other clinical symptoms.

ASO and siRNA strategies have been intensively studied on DM1 cellular models such as patient fibroblasts and mouse or drosophila models containing up to 1,000 CTG triplets in the DMPK gene and in clinical trial with a gapmer ASO containing constrained ethyl (cEt) locked nucleic acid (LNA). A recent clinical trial was initiated in 2022 with DYNE-101, a muscle membrane antigen-binding fragment antibody (FAB) conjugated to an ASO to enable targeted muscle tissue delivery.

The multiple strategies displayed in Figure 10.9 illustrate that DM1 represents a model disease case where multiple RNA drug interventions can be envisioned, either separately or in combination. Since MBNL proteins are sequestered by poly-CTG DMPK nuclear foci, the use of ASO or siRNA carrying a poly-ACG triplet may lead to DMPK nuclear foci cleavage and degradation. Alternatively, an ASO can also function as a steric blocker of MBNL binding, thus releasing the necessary amount of MBNL to restore the adult phenotype splicing pattern (Figures 10.9(A and B)).

A second strategy is to target the miRNA (miR)23b, which has been shown to negatively control MBNL expression. Thus, the administration of a blocker ASO complementary to (miR)23b would up-regulate MBNL expression and potentially compensate for the sequestration of MBNL by

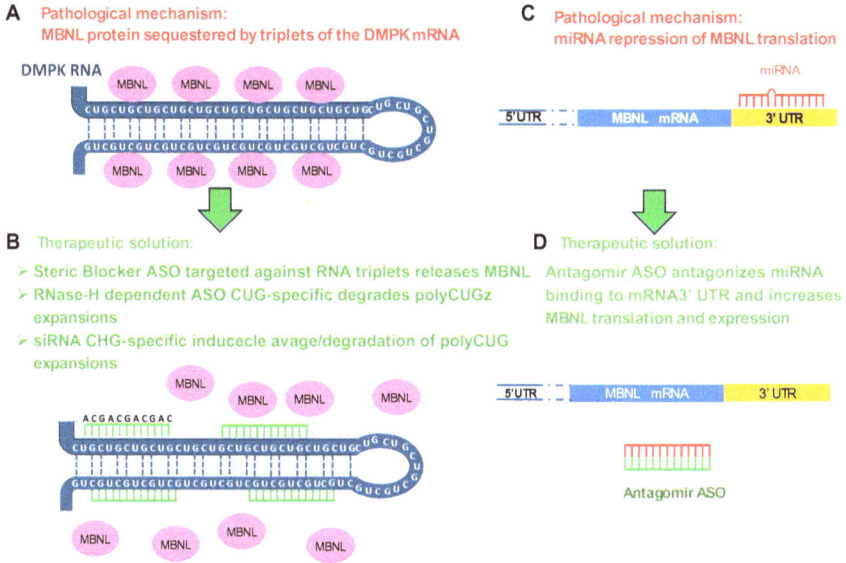

**A** Pathological mechanism:
MBNL protein sequestered by triplets of the DMPK mRNA

**B** Therapeutic solution:

➢ Steric Blocker ASO targeted against RNA triplets releases MBNL
➢ RNase-H dependent ASO CUG-specific degrades polyCUGz expansions
➢ siRNA CHG-specific inducecle avage/degradation of polyCUG expansions

**C** Pathological mechanism:
miRNA repression of MBNL translation

**D** Therapeutic solution:
Antagomir ASO antagonizes miRNA binding to mRNA 3' UTR and increases MBNL translation and expression

**Figure 10.9.** Different ASO- and siRNA-based strategies against Myotonic Dystrophy Type 1. (A) MBNL proteins are sequestered by nuclear foci formed by mRNA from the poly-CTG DMPK variant. (B) Poly-ACG ASO or siRNA lead to DMPK mRNA cleavage and nuclear foci degradation. Alternatively, they can also function as steric blockers of MBNL binding to the foci, thus releasing the necessary amount of MBNL required for restoring the adult phenotype splicing pattern. (C, D) Since the miRNA (miR)23b has been shown to repress MBNL expression, the administration of antagomir-23b antagonizes the miRNA (miR)23b, which increases MBNL expression, thus compensating for the sequestration of MBNL by variant DMPK mRNA.

variant DMPK mRNA (Figures 10.9(C and D)). Finally, since MBNL sequestering and lack of availability induces mis-splicing toward the fetal phenotype of various proteins, splice corrector ASOs, similar to the one described in Figure 10.7 for SMA, represent an appealing strategy to restore the expression of the adult form of the critical mis-spliced proteins. Such a downstream approach has been successfully reported using a morpholino ASO to restore the muscle chloride channel. This was achieved in electroporated muscle fibers or using ultrasound-enhanced delivery of morpholinos with bubble liposomes (see Chapter 7).

# Bibliography

Aartsma-Rus A, Fokkema I, Verschuuren J, Ginjaar I, van Deutekom J, van Ommen GJ, den Dunnen JT. Theoretic applicability of antisense-mediated exon skipping for Duchenne muscular dystrophy mutations. *Hum Mutat.* 2009 Mar;30(3):293–9. doi: 10.1002/humu.20918.

Amantana A, Iversen PL. Pharmacokinetics and biodistribution of phosphorodi-amidate morpholino antisense oligomers. *Curr Opin Pharmacol.* 2005 Oct;5(5):550–5. doi: 10.1016/j.coph.2005.07.001.

Bennett CF, Krainer AR, Cleveland DW. Antisense oligonucleotide therapies for neurodegenerative diseases. *Annu Rev Neurosci.* 2019 Jul 8;42:385–406. doi: 10.1146/annurev-neuro-070918-050501.

Brunet de Courssou JB, Durr A, Adams D, Corvol JC, Mariani LL. Antisense therapies in neurological diseases. *Brain.* 2022 Apr 29;145(3):816–31. doi: 10.1093/brain/awab423.

Burlet P, Bürglen L, Clermont O, Lefebvre S, Viollet L, Munnich A, Melki J. Large scale deletions of the 5q13 region are specific to Werdnig-Hoffmann disease. *J Med Genet.* 1996 Apr;33(4):281–3. doi: 10.1136/jmg.33.4.281.

Chen B, Gong Y, Zhou T. The impact of nusinersen and risdiplam on motor function for spinal muscular atrophy type 2 and 3: a meta-analysis. *J Coll Physicians Surg Pak.* 2024 Aug;34(8):948–55. doi: 10.29271/jcpsp.2024.08.948.

Codron P, Cassereau J, Vourc'h P. InFUSing antisense oligonucleotides for treating ALS. *Trends Mol Med.* 2022 Apr;28(4):253–4. doi: 10.1016/j.molmed.2022.02.006.

Crooke ST, Liang XH, Baker BF, Crooke RM. Antisense technology: A review. *J Biol Chem.* 2021 Jan-Jun;296:100416. doi: 10.1016/j.jbc.2021.100416.

Debacker AJ, Voutila J, Catley M, Blakey D, Habib N. Delivery of oligonucleotides to the liver with GalNAc: from research to registered therapeutic drug. *Mol Ther.* 2020 Aug 5;28(8):1759–71. doi: 10.1016/j.ymthe.2020.06.015.

Dyck PJB, Coelho T, Waddington Cruz M, Brannagan TH 3rd, Khella S, Karam C, Berk JL, Polydefkis MJ, *et al.* Neuropathy symptom and change: inotersen treatment of hereditary transthyretin amyloidosis. *Muscle Nerve.* 2020 Oct;62(4):509–15. doi: 10.1002/mus.27023.

Eckstein F. Phosphorothioates, essential components of therapeutic oligonucleotides. *Nucleic Acid Ther.* 2014 Dec;24(6):374–87. doi: 10.1089/nat.2014.0506.

Fattal E, Bochot A. Ocular delivery of nucleic acids: antisense oligonucleotides, aptamers and siRNA. *Adv Drug Deliv Rev*. 2006 Nov 15;58(11):1203–23. doi: 10.1016/j.addr.2006.07.020.

Furdon PJ, Dominski Z, Kole R. RNase H cleavage of RNA hybridized to oligonucleotides containing methylphosphonate, phosphorothioate and phosphodiester bonds. *Nucleic Acids Res*. 1989 Nov 25;17(22):9193–204. doi: 10.1093/nar/17.22.9193.

Gennemark P, Walter K, Clemmensen N, Rekić D, Nilsson CAM, Knöchel J, Höltta M, Wernevik L, *et al*. An oral antisense oligonucleotide for PCSK9 inhibition. *Sci Transl Med*. 2021 May 12;13(593):eabe9117. doi: 10.1126/scitranslmed.abe9117.

Giess D, Erdos J, Wild C. An updated systematic review on spinal muscular atrophy patients treated with nusinersen, onasemnogene abeparvovec (at least 24 months), risdiplam (at least 12 months) or combination therapies. *Eur J Paediatr Neurol*. 2024 Jul;51:84–92. doi: 10.1016/j.ejpn.2024.06.004.

Goyenvalle A, Vulin A, Fougerousse F, Leturcq F, Kaplan JC, Garcia L, Danos O. Rescue of dystrophic muscle through U7 snRNA-mediated exon skipping. *Science*. 2004 Dec 3;306(5702):1796–9. doi: 10.1126/science.1104297.

Goyenvalle A, Leumann C, Garcia L. Therapeutic potential of tricyclo-DNA antisense oligonucleotides. *J Neuromuscul Dis*. 2016 May 27;3(2):157–67. doi: 10.3233/JND-160146.

Hagenacker T, Maggi L, Coratti G, Youn B, Raynaud S, Paradis AD, Mercuri E. Effectiveness of nusinersen in adolescents and adults with spinal muscular atrophy: Systematic review and meta-analysis. *Neurol Ther*. 2024 Oct;13(5): 1483–504. doi: 10.1007/s40120-024-00653-2.

Holm A, Hansen SN, Klitgaard H, Kauppinen S. Clinical advances of RNA therapeutics for treatment of neurological and neuromuscular diseases. *RNA Biol*. 2022;19(1):594–608. doi: 10.1080/15476286.2022.2066334.

Khvorova A, Watts JK. The chemical evolution of oligonucleotide therapies of clinical utility. *Nat Biotechnol*. 2017 Mar;35(3):238–48. doi: 10.1038/nbt.3765.

Nguyen Q, Yokota T. Degradation of toxic RNA in myotonic dystrophy using gapmer antisense oligonucleotides. *Methods Mol Biol*. 2020;2176:99–109. doi: 10.1007/978-1-0716-0771-8_7.

Pang J, Guo Q, Lu Z. The catalytic mechanism, metal dependence, substrate specificity, and biodiversity of ribonuclease H. *Front Microbiol*. 2022 Nov 21;13:1034811. doi: 10.3389/fmicb.2022.1034811.

Renneberg D, Bouliong E, Reber U, Schümperli D, Leumann CJ. Antisense properties of tricyclo-DNA. *Nucleic Acids Res*. 2002 Jul 1;30(13):2751–7. doi: 10.1093/nar/gkf412.

Shen W, De Hoyos CL, Sun H, Vickers TA, Liang XH, Crooke ST. Acute hepatotoxicity of 2' fluoro-modified 5-10-5 gapmer phosphorothioate oligonucleotides in mice correlates with intracellular protein binding and the loss of DBHS proteins. *Nucleic Acids Res*. 2018 Mar 16;46(5):2204–17. doi: 10.1093/nar/gky060.

Singh NK, Singh NN, Androphy EJ, Singh RN. Splicing of a critical exon of human survival motor neuron is regulated by a unique silencer element located in the last intron. *Mol Cell Biol*. 2006 Feb;26(4):1333–46. doi: 10.1128/MCB.26.4.1333-1346.2006.

Stein CA. Eteplirsen approved for Duchenne muscular dystrophy: the FDA faces a difficult choice. *Mol Ther*. 2016 Nov;24(11):1884–5. doi: 10.1038/mt.2016.188.

Stephenson ML, Zamecnik PC. Inhibition of Rous sarcoma viral RNA translation by a specific oligodeoxyribonucleotide. *Proc Natl Acad Sci U S A*. 1978 Jan;75(1):285–8. doi: 10.1073/pnas.75.1.285.

Wirth B, Brichta L, Schrank B, Lochmüller H, Blick S, Baasner A, Heller R. Mildly affected patients with spinal muscular atrophy are partially protected by an increased SMN2 copy number. *Hum Genet*. 2006 May;119(4):422–8. doi: 10.1007/s00439-006-0156-7.

Zhang L, Liang XH, De Hoyos CL, Migawa M, Nichols JG, Freestone G, Tian J, Seth PP, Crooke ST. The combination of mesyl-phosphoramidate internucleotide linkages and 2'-O-methyl in selected positions in the antisense oligonucleotide enhances the performance of RNaseH1 active PS-ASOs. *Nucleic Acid Ther*. 2022 Oct;32(5):401–11. doi: 10.1089/nat.2022.0005.

# Chapter 11

# RNA Silencing and Small Interfering RNA

## 11.1  Mechanism of RNA Interference and of siRNA

As an alternative to the antisense approach, the second strategy to suppress a targeted mRNA in a sequence-specific manner makes use of the RNA interference process (RNAi). RNA interference is a natural microRNA-mediated process (miRNA) that is central to the post-transcriptional silencing regulation of many basic cellular and developmental programs. This process is schematized in Figure 11.1.

The miRNAs derive from regions of RNA transcripts that fold back on themselves to form short hairpins whose main characteristic is the presence of one or several mismatches in the self-complementary sequence. The miRNA maturation basic steps comprise the transcription by RNA polymerase II of a primary miRNA (pri-miRNA). The pri-miRNA, is processed in the cell nucleus into an approximately 70 nucleotide pre-miRNA by the microprocessor complex, Drosha/DGCR8. The microprocessor complex subunit, DiGeorge-syndrome critical region 8 (DGCR8), contains an RNA-binding domain which stabilizes the primary miRNA for processing by the second microprocessor subunit, Drosha, an RNase III enzyme. The pri-miRNA is cleaved by the Drosha/DGCR8 complex into a characteristic stem-loop structure known as a pre-miRNA.

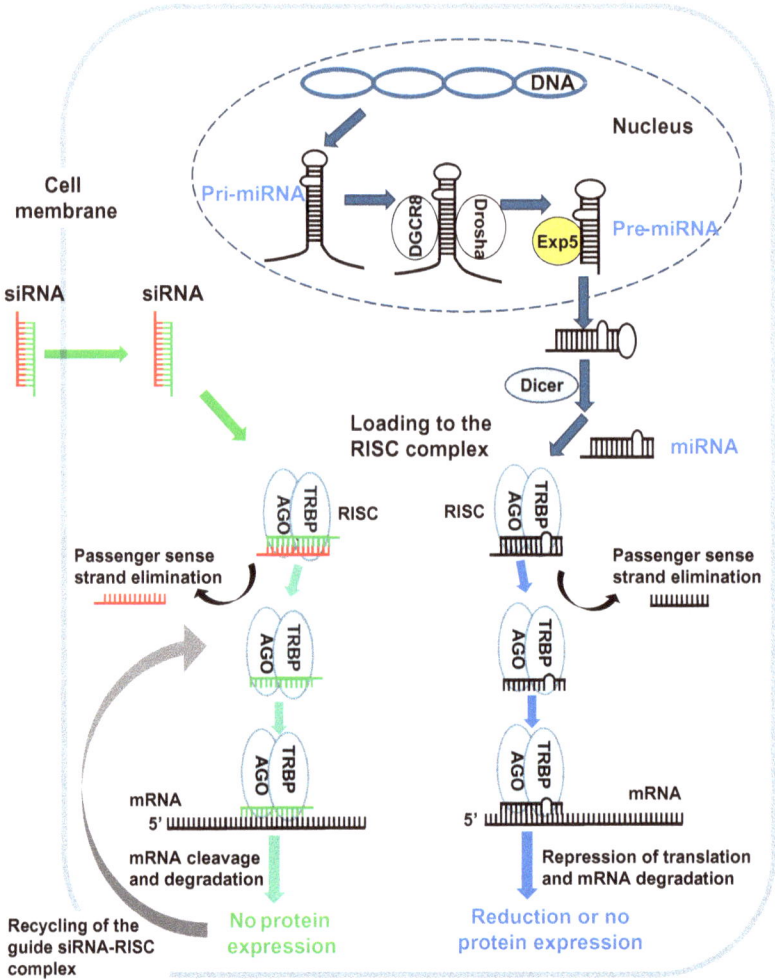

**Figure 11.1.** Mechanism of miRNA and siRNA action. (top center and right side): Blue arrows represent the canonical miRNA maturation and mechanism of action pathway. Transcription leads to a pri-miRNA, which folds into a small hairpin RNA with one or several mismatches. The pri-miRNA is processed by Drosha and DGCR8 to a pre-miRNA. After association with exportin 5, the pre-miRNA is transported through the nuclear envelope by a process dependent on the small GTPase ran-GTP. The pre-miRNA is finally processed by the Dicer endoribonuclease (a class III RNase), which deletes the hairpin loop. This generates an RNA duplex made of a passenger and a guide strand. After miRNA homoduplex association with the RISC complex composed of protein TRBP and the argonaute-2 nuclease, the passenger strand is eliminated. The RISC/guide strand

Pre-miRNAs possess a hairpin structure with stems containing interspersed mismatches and are exported across the nuclear envelope into the cytosol by binding to exportin 5.

The next step occurs through a cytoplasmic process where the riboendonuclease Dicer mediates the cleavage of the pre-miRNA at the base of the stem (hence removing the terminal loop) to form the double-stranded mature miRNA duplex. Then, the RNA-induced silencing complex (RISC) eliminates the miRNA sense passenger strand and retains binding to the antisense strand. This antisense strand is also called the "guide" strand because it allows the specific binding of the RISC complex to the complementary Watson–Crick sequence on the targeted mRNA. The RISC complex is composed of the protein TRBP and the argonaute-2 nuclease (Ago).

Natural miRNA target sites tend to cluster in the mRNA 3' untranslated region, although other miRNA sites have been found in different mRNA regions. The binding of miRNA/RISC leads to the repression of mRNA translation and, in certain proportions, to mRNA cleavage by Ago. The presence of mismatches favors translation repression; however, in a minority of cases, the absence of mismatches induces complete mRNA cleavage.

---

**Figure 11.1.**   (*Continued*) complex binds to the target mRNA at the 5' non-translated region, inducing a steric blockage of ribosome entry and translation. In some instances, miRNA binding can also lead to mRNA cleavage and degradation; however, a mismatch usually decreases the probability of this occurring. Alternatively, a gene expression cassette coding a small hairpin RNA (shRNA) is administered either as a plasmid or via a viral gene delivery vector. The shRNA transcript is then processed, like the miRNA. However, no mismatches are introduced, which leads to fully efficient mRNA degradation and silencing. (left side): siRNA mechanism (green arrows). A double-strand synthetic siRNA with no mismatch is administered to the cells. All action takes place in the cytosol. After siRNA binding to the RISC complex composed of protein TRBP and the argonaute-2 nuclease, the passenger strand is eliminated. The guide strand complexed to RISC binds to the target mRNA. The target sequence is generally chosen within the translated region. Because of the complete siRNA matching with the mRNA target sequence, argonaute-2 is now able to cleave the target mRNA with great efficiency. After mRNA cleavage and elimination, the RISC/guide siRNA complex can bind and cleave another mRNA (gray arrow).

For therapeutic use of this endogenous mRNA degradation process, two strategies have been employed. In the first one, an expression cassette DNA containing a short gene encoding self-complementary mRNA is delivered to the cells. The resulting mRNA transcript forms a short hairpin (shRNA), which is processed by the Drosha/DGCR8 complex in the same manner as pri-miRNA. The shRNAs possess a completely base-paired 19–29 nt stem, ensuring Dicer cleavage step to produce the final siRNA. The resulting siRNA duplex has symmetric, 2-nucleotide 3' overhangs with a 19–21 base-pair region. It associates with the RISC ribonucleoprotein complex, leading to the complete RNA interference process and targeted mRNA degradation. In most published cases, shRNA transgenes are delivered using either an AAV or a lentiviral gene delivery vector. The shRNA technique is widely used in the laboratory stage, since it is available through standard expertise and ensures continuous intracellular shRNA messenger and siRNA production, as well as efficient and selective silencing.

The second RNA interference therapeutic strategy uses exogenous siRNAs, which are constituted of chemically synthesized double-strand short oligoribonucleotides and are fully complementary 20–23 base pair ribonucleotides. As shown in Figures 11.1 and 11.2, the siRNA mechanism of action also involves RISC. The siRNAs are administered as two-strand, perfectly matched Watson–Crick homoduplexes. One "antisense" strand, which is also called the "guide" strand, is complementary to a sequence of the targeted mRNA. In contrary to the microRNA mechanism, no mismatch is tolerated between the guide strand and the targeted mRNA sequence. In addition, both 3' ends possess two supplementary overhanging non-hybridized nucleotides.

The chemistry of such a synthetic siRNA homoduplex is designed to be recognized by the RISC nucleoprotein complex, which dissociates the sense siRNA strand. As with miRNAs, the RISC complex is then guided by the antisense strand to bind to the complementary sequence on the targeted mRNA, leading to mRNA nucleolytic cleavage and degradation (Figures 11.1 and 11.2). Since the guide sense is designed to perfectly

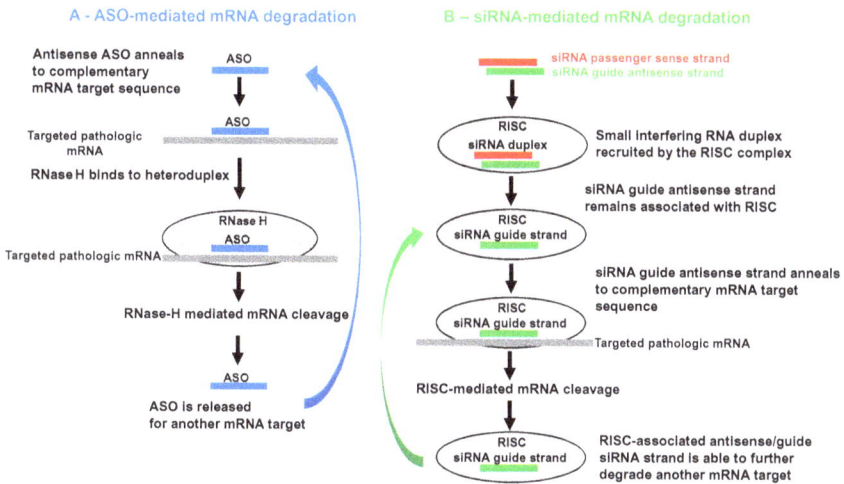

**Figure 11.2.**   ASO versus siRNA mediated mRNA degradation. (A) ASO deoxynucleotide (blue rod) hybridizes with target mRNA. The deoxyASO/mRNA heteroduplex is scouted and recognized by RNase H. RNase H then degrades mRNA. This causes the dissociation of ASO from both mRNA and RNase H. The ASO is then free to scout another mRNA (blue curved arrow). (B) Double-stranded homoduplex siRNA is recruited by the RISC complex. The passenger "sense" strand (red rod) is released from the complex. The antisense guide strand (green rod) remains positioned within the RISC complex and stabilizes it on the targeted complementary mRNA sequence through fully complementary Watson–Crick hybridization. This induces mRNA cleavage. The cleaved mRNA is dissociated, and the RISC/guide siRNA complex can associate and cleave another mRNA (green curved arrow).

match its complementary sequence on the targeted mRNA, the Ago-mediated mRNA cleavage is complete.

Once this occurs, the RISC/guide siRNA complex can be used again to target and cleave another pathologic mRNA. This recycling process, associated with optimized chemistry, enables high siRNA metabolic stability and ensures a prolonged duration of action. Indeed, *in vivo* effects have been reported for the most recently developed siRNA drugs with a spectacular duration of action surpassing six months following a single administration.

## 11.2   Comparison Between ASO and siRNA Properties

The ASO and siRNA characteristics and specificities listed in Table 11.1 are responsible for marked differences in physicochemical and pharmacokinetic properties, which dictate different required chemical optimization, depending on the nature of the drug and the targeted tissue. A single-stranded ASO is more flexible and accessible to endonuclease and thus necessitates complete protection of each phosphodiester linkage against nucleases. On the other hand, a double-helix siRNA shows more resistance in its internal phosphodiester linkages. A single-stranded ASO also displays the hydrophobic moieties from its nucleic bases, which is not the case for double-helical siRNA. Hence, ASOs will bind to plasma proteins such as albumin, which leads to a longer circulation time and enhanced biodistribution to tissues. On the contrary, natural siRNAs are rapidly eliminated by kidney filtration and need a delivery vector, such as a lipid

**Table 11.1.**   Comparison between ASO and siRNA drugs.

| ASO | siRNA |
|---|---|
| Single stranded | Double stranded |
| 14–20 bases — linear deoxynucleotide | 21–23 base pairs RNA |
| Flexible with ~ 1 nm width | Rigid duplex ~ 2 nm diameter |
| Single-stranded nature requires full backbone modification with phosphorothioate (PS) linkages to protect from nucleases | Double-stranded nature ensures relative protection against nucleases |
| Design must retain ribose sugars moieties in the seed center sequence to allow RNase H activity | Ribose sugars can be modified to a certain limit with respect to argonaute efficiency |
| Sugar modifications are tolerated only on wings of a gapmer | Sugar modifications tolerated |
| Hydrophobic surfaces accessible for protein interactions allow binding to plasma proteins such as albumin and increase blood circulation and biodistribution to tissues | Little exposed hydrophobic surface since aromatic bases are paired and buried in duplex |
| | Hydrophilic surface causes rapid kidney clearance unless targeted to a specific tissue or organ |

nanoparticle (LNP) formulation or a functional targeting moiety directed toward an extracellular receptor.

Other differences between ASOs and siRNAs originate from the fact that only binding to the target mRNA is required to achieve ASO function as steric blocker, while for mRNA degradation the catalytic activity of RNase H (for ASOs) and of argonaute-2 (for siRNAs) must be maintained (Figure 11.2). From the comparison in Figure 11.2, it appears that the recycling process is simpler and presumably faster with siRNA, since the guide antisense strand remains associated with the RISC system for binding to each new mRNA target, while with ASO the recruitment of a new RNase H is required after mRNA degradation. Thus, the catalytically induced mRNA degradation represents a one-step molecular recognition process for the RISC/siRNA complex, while it is a two-step molecular recognition process for the ASO/RNase H process.

Finally, it is generally considered that ASOs can block or cleave both pre-mRNA and mRNA either in the nucleus or in the cytosol, while siRNA ensures the degradation of mature mRNA only in the cytosol. This represents a crucial difference for diseases caused by the nuclear aggregation of variant mRNA, such as Myotonic Dystrophy Type 1 (MD1) (Section 10.10 of Chapter 10). This concern is, however, a disputed point because several siRNAs and shRNAs have been shown to lead to nuclear foci degradation in MD1 cellular and animal models, thus suggesting that the RISC-induced cleavage and subsequent degradation could also occur in the nucleus.

## 11.3  Chemical and Delivery Optimization of siRNAs

In contrast to ASOs, which might be efficient as steric blockers without concomitant nuclease activity, the efficacy of siRNAs strictly depends on argonaute-2 nucleolytic activity. As for RNase H-dependent ASOs, the modifications introduced into the guide antisense siRNA strand to increase its metabolic stability are limited and must be finely optimized. More freedom for modifications is allowed on the passenger sense strand, which is not involved in RISC-mediated nuclease activity. An additional constraint to consider is limiting the innate immune response induced by natural RNA duplexes, which has initially represented a major obstacle in the development of siRNA technology.

A mapping of the functional domains of a typical siRNA provides guidance on where chemical diversity can be introduced (Figure 11.3(A)). While most siRNA designs are based on a non-covalent two-strand double helix (Figures 11.3(A and B)), corresponding to the clinically approved RNA drugs as of 2024, other concepts have been proposed and shown to possess promising properties, at least at the preclinical level, such as di-siRNA composed of two double-helical siRNAs made of one double-sized passenger strand and two guide strands (Figure 11.3(C)). An interesting siRNA geometry is that of a nicked hairpin (Figure 11.3(D)). While the guide antisense strand is of 22 bases canonical length, the sense passenger strand is longer (36 bases), and it auto-hybridizes itself through a G-C rich sequence (GCAGCC hybridized to CGUCGG) to form a GAAA loop at its extremity. A nick in the hairpin structure is located between the sense and antisense strands. Targeting moieties, such as GalNac sugars, have been linked to the GAAA loop, thus providing a high tetravalent sugar moiety for targeting liver hepatocytes.

The presence of a 5' phosphate on the siRNA guide strand is an essential factor for entry into the RISC complex and loading onto the Ago2 nuclease. Stable phosphate analogs, such as phosphonates, have been introduced with a strong enhancement effect (Figure 11.3(A)). A non-cleavable targeting moiety can be linked to the passenger strand. With a tri-antennary GalNac targeting head which binds to the hepatocyte asialoglycoprotein receptor, a dramatic increase in liver uptake and silencing efficiency has been observed, leading to several months of silencing effect after a single dose. This represents one of the most exciting perspectives of siRNA therapeutics for liver-associated diseases (see Section 6.8 of Chapter 6).

While 2'-fluoro ribose modification is well tolerated by the RISC machinery, phosphodiester linkage substitution by phosphorothioate can only be introduced in a limited number of nucleotides, which is outside the seed region and cleavage site. Similarly, sugar modifications such as 2'-OMe or LNA are more tolerated on the passenger strand, and they

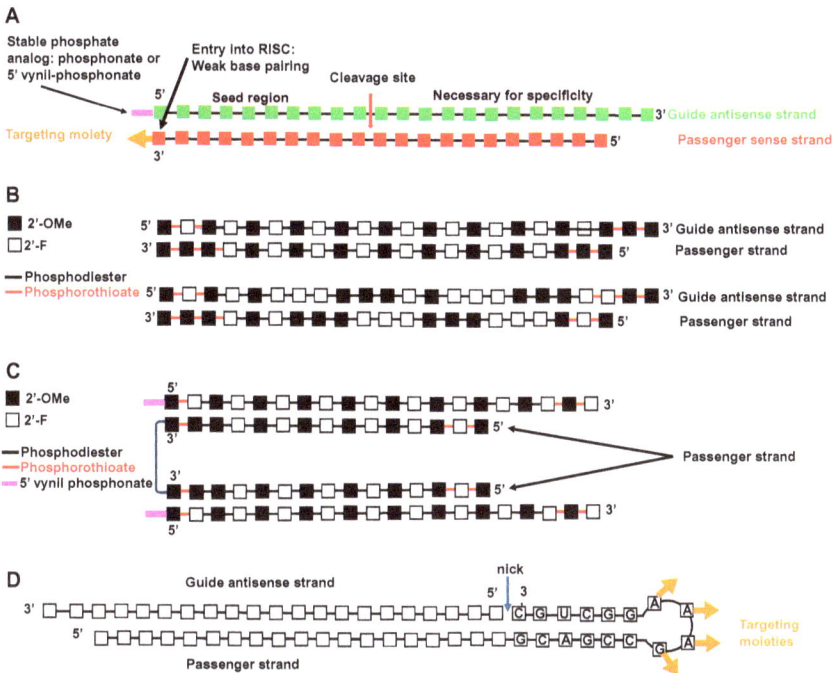

**Figure 11.3.** Different published siRNA geometries. (A) The siRNA functional regions. More modifications are tolerated on the passenger strand (red squares), which is not involved in argonaute-2-mediated mRNA cleavage. A targeting moiety can be covalently linked to the 3' end of the passenger strand (orange arrow). A stable phosphonate resistant to dephosphorylation enzymes can be included instead of a phosphate (velvet rod) at the 5' end of the guide antisense siRNA (green square). Both are necessary and compatible for the binding of the guide strand to the RISC complex. Fewer modifications are allowed in the seed region of the guide siRNA strand (nucleotides 2–8). An optimized guide strand must contain a flexible 5' end (which can be obtained by lowering base pairing and facilitates capture by the RISC complex), a high-affinity "seed" region, which drives the initial base pairing between the guide strand and mRNA target, and a lower-affinity 3'-region required for cleaved mRNA release. (B) Frequently used siRNAs are made resistant to exonucleases by 2–3 terminal phosphorothioate linkages on both 3' and 5' terminals of each strand. Modified sugars 2'-OMe and 2'-fluoro have led to siRNAs that are highly resistant to nuclease and are of improved bioavailability and high binding affinity for the RISC complex. This leads to an unprecedented duration of action which can reach up to six months or more after a single administration due to the recycling mechanism displayed in Figures 11.1 and 11.2. (C) Schematic diagram of a di-siRNA. (D) In this presented geometry, the antisense strand is of 22 nucleotides canonical length, while the sense passenger strand is much longer (36 nucleotides), and it auto-hybridizes through a GC-rich sequence (GCAGCC hybridized to GGCUGC) to form a GAAA loop at its extremity.

are favored at the 5' end because they block passenger strand entry into the RISC complex and consequently favor RISC-exclusive loading with the guide strand.

Two typical popular siRNA geometries are displayed in Figure 11.3(B). In the upper siRNA, 2'-fluoro and 2'-OMe are intercalated and face each other to obtain a canonical alpha helix geometry. In the second more widely used formula, stretches of three consecutive 2'-fluoro and 2'-OMe nucleotides are present and frequently face each other. Two to three phosphorothioate linkages are introduced at the 5' and 3' ends of both strands, which ensures sufficient metabolic stability against exonucleases. Another backbone modification has been recently introduced in the form of a divalent siRNA, in which two passenger moieties are covalently linked (Figure 11.3(C)). These di-siRNAs display a favorable distribution in the central nervous system and exhibit promising efficacy in neurodegenerative disease models in rodents and non-human primates.

While the maximum number of 2'fluoro must be controlled because of potential liver toxicity, other modifications have proved useful, such as 5' carbon pyrimidines. Moreover, using a systematic iterative screening technology, it has been shown that optimizing the positioning of 2'-deoxy-2'-fluoro and 2'-O-methyl ribose across both strands enhances metabolic stability. This could be obtained with a low 2'-deoxy-2'-fluoro content.

Numerous formulations have been proposed to improve siRNA pharmacokinetics, such as LNPs (described in Section 6.7 of Chapter 6). LNPs have proven their efficacy in targeting the liver *in vivo*, leading to the clinically approved *patisiran* siRNA drug for treating transthyretin amyloidosis. While liver targeting is presently well mastered using either LNP or the GalNac technologies (see Section 6.8 of Chapter 6), challenges remain for other organs, particularly the brain; however, progress is being made in terms of oral and ocular delivery as well as intravenous delivery to inflammatory sites.

The following sections illustrate the above concepts by describing a selection of typical examples of siRNA approaches for treating multiple disorders, for which marketing approval or very promising results have been obtained. Since any genetic disease might benefit from anti-mRNA siRNA technology, this cannot be exhaustively described here.

## 11.4 Overview of siRNAs Therapeutic Applications

Ideally, any disease in which a pathological gene can be safely silenced is a reasonable candidate for siRNA therapy. However, insufficient delivery to target cells and tissue represents the main challenge to the wide extension of this technology. Nevertheless, the list of applications currently being actively developed by pharmaceutical or biotech companies is already striking given the relatively recent introduction of this technology, and this list increases at a fast rate. Table 11.2 presents a non-exhaustive list of siRNA applications in the clinic or in development, together with the targeted gene.

**Table 11.2.** Examples of siRNAs approved (Ap) or in clinical development.

| Disease | Targeted gene | Tissue | Drug denomination |
|---|---|---|---|
| **Rare genetic diseases** | | | |
| Acute hepatic porphyria | Hepatic delta aminolevulinate synthase 1 | Liver | Givosiran (Ap) |
| ATTR amyloidosis | Hepatic mutant transthyretin | Liver | Patisiran, vutrisiran (Ap) |
| Hemophilia and rare bleeding disorders | Hepatic antithrombin | Liver | Fitusiran (Ap) |
| Primary hyperoxaluria type I or 1/2 | Hepatic hydroxyacid oxidase 1 | Liver | Lumasiran (Ap) |
| Primary hyperoxaluria type I or 1/2 | Hepatic lactate dehydrogenase | Liver | Nedosiran (Ap) |
| Alpha-antitrypsin deficiency | Mutant alpha antitrypsin | Liver | Fazirsiran (ARO-AAT) / ALN-AAT02 / belcesiran |
| Alport syndrome | MicroRNA-21 (miR-21) | Liver | RG-012 |
| Beta-thalassemia-myeloblastic syndrome-iron loading anemia | TMPRSS6 matriptase 2 (hepcidin modulator) | Liver | SLN-124 |

*(Continued)*

**Table 11.2.** (*Continued*)

| Disease | Targeted gene | Tissue | Drug denomination |
|---|---|---|---|
| Cystic fibrosis | Epithelial sodium channel ENaC | Lung | ARO-ENaC |
| Immunoglobin A nephropathy | C5 component of the complement | Liver | Cemdisiran |
| **Infectious diseases** | | | |
| Chronic HBV infection | All HBV transcripts | Liver | ARB-001467 / VIR-2218 |
| Chronic hepatitis B infection | All HBV transcripts | Liver | A JNJ3989 / ARB-729 / DCR-HBVS |
| **Eye diseases** | | | |
| Diabetic macular edema | Vascular endothelial growth factor VEGF | Eye | PF-655 |
| Dry eye disease | TRPV1 receptor | Eye | Tivanisiran (SYL1001) |
| Glaucoma | VEGF | Eye | Bamosiran |
| Non arteritic anterior ischaemic optic neuropathy | Pro-apoptotic protein caspase 2 | Eye | QPI-1007 |
| Oculopharyngeal muscular dystrophy (OPMD) | Mutant PABPN1 gene | Eye muscle | BB-301 |
| **Cardiovascular** | | | |
| Cardiovascular disease — hypercholesterolemia | Apolipoprotein a (liver) | Liver | AMG890 — olpasiran |
| Complement C3 | Complement component 5 (C5) | Liver | SLN-500 |
| Dyslipidemia — hypertriglyceridemia | Apolipoprotein C-III (liver) | Liver | ARO-APOC3 / plozasiran |
| Heart failure | MicroRNA-92a (blood vessels) | Blood vessels | MRG-110 |
| Hypercholesterolemia | Hepatic PCSK9 | Liver | Inclisiran |

**Table 11.2.** (*Continued*)

| Disease | Targeted gene | Tissue | Drug denomination |
|---|---|---|---|
| Hypertension | Angiotensin II (liver) | Liver | Zilebesiran (ALN-AGT01) |
| Lp(a) for cardiovascular diseases | Lipoprotein (a) (liver) | Liver | SLN-360 |
| **Cancer and overgrowth syndromes** | | | |
| Advanced solid tumors | VEGF-A and Kinase Spindle Pole (KSP) | Tumor | ALN-VSP02 |
| Advanced solid tumors | Protein kinase N3 | Endothelium | Atu027 |
| Advanced solid tumors | Polo-like kinase protein | Tumor | TKM-PLK1 |
| Hypertrophic scars / keloid | TGFβ1 and COX2 | Scar; keloid | Cotsiranib |
| Hypertrophic scars / keloid | Connective tissue growth factor CTGF | Scar; keloid | RXI-109 / BMT101 / OLX10010 |
| Melanoma | PD-1 mRNA | Tumor | PH-762 |
| Pancreatic cancer | KRASG12D oncogene | Tumor | SiG120 / KRS G12D |
| Renal cell carcinoma | HIF2alpha — hypoxia induced factor 2 | Tumor | Arrow-HIF2 |
| Solid tumors | EphA2 — ephrin type-A receptor 2 | Tumor | EphA2-DOPC |
| Various cancers | TIGIT | NK cells | PH-804 |
| **Others** | | | |
| Prophylaxis of acute kidney injury | p53 | Kidney | Tepresiran |
| Idiopathic pulmonary or hepatic fibrosis | HSP47 | Lung or liver | ND-L02-s0201 |
| Non-alcoholic steatohepatitis NASH | HSD17B13 — hydroxysteroid 17-beta dehydrogenase 13 | Liver | ALN-HSD |
| Pachyonychia congenita | Keratin K6a | Skin | TD101 |

## 11.5 Applications of siRNAs Delivered to the Liver

### 11.5.1 *Transthyretin hereditary amyloidosis*

*Patisiran*, sold under the brand name Onpattro, has been clinically approved for the treatment of polyneuropathy in people with hereditary transthyretin-mediated amyloidosis, a fatal rare disease estimated to affect 50,000 people worldwide. It is the first siRNA-based drug that has been clinically approved. It silences the production of mutated transthyretin in genetic hereditary transthyretin amyloidosis (hATTR). It is formulated in an LNP and IV administered, leading to a strong accumulation in the liver by binding to the ApoE receptor (Section 6.7 of Chapter 6).

The antisense guide strand formula is A-U-G-G-A-A-Um-A-C-U-C-U-U-G-G-U-Um-A-C-dT-dT). It is complexed with the complementary passenger sense strand (G-Um-A-A-Cm-Cm-A-A-G-A-G-Um-A-Um-Um-Cm-Cm-A-Um-dT-dT (A, adenosine; C, cytidine; G, guanosine; U, uridine; Cm, 2'-O-methylcytidine; Um, 2'-O-methyluridine; dT, thymidine). Thus, *patisiran* bears eleven 2'-O-methylated pyrimidines, which increases its lipophilicity. All inter-ribose linkages are phosphodiester. The structural formula is displayed in Figure 11.4.

*Vutrisiran* (Amvuttra™) is a subcutaneously administered transthyretin-specific siRNA, developed in a second step for hATTR. *Vutrisiran* was clinically approved in 2022 for the treatment of human transthyretin

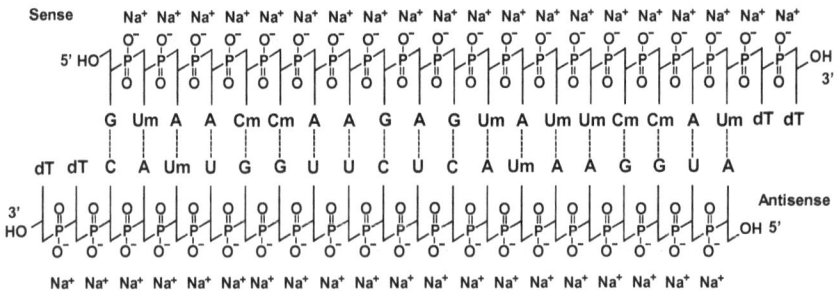

**Figure 11.4.** Structural formula of *patisiran*. A: adenosine; G: guanosine; U: uridine; Cm: 2'-O-methylcytidine; Um: 2'-O-methyluridine; dt: thymidine.

amyloidosis with polyneuropathy in adults, after fast-track designation in 2020 in view of the very promising efficacy of this RNA drug.

The *vutrisiran* sequence was designed to bind to a conserved sequence on all TTR mRNA variants. Because *vutrisiran* is administered as a naked siRNA, i.e., not associated with a lipid nanoparticle delivery system, the drug must be metabolically protected and targeted to hepatocytes. Nuclease resistance has been achieved by introducing significantly more modifications in *vutrisiran* than in *patisiran*. Indeed, while *patrisiran* contains only eleven 2'-O-Me nucleotides and only phosphodiester linkages, *vutrisiran* is a heavily modified siRNA with six phosphorothioate linkages at the end of each strand, 35 nucleotides carrying a 2'-OMe ribose, and nine nucleotides modified with a 2'F ribose. Thus, the two *vutrisiran* strands (one of 21 nt and one of 23 nt) are fully modified. Optimization of the number and respective positions of these modifications has been performed to reduce toxicity, particularly hepatotoxicity.

The striking property of *vutrisiran* is its exceptional capacity to target hepatocytes through a trigalactosyl moiety branched to the passenger sense strand, which binds with high affinity to the asialoglycoprotein receptor (Figure 11.5 and Section 6.8 of Chapter 6).

The improved metabolic stability of *vutrisiran*, along with the very potent targeting efficacy of its tri-Gal-Nac, leads to its exceptional intrinsic efficacy. This is demonstrated by the therapeutic efficacy of very low doses and the exceptionally long duration of action, since a quarterly regimen is sufficient to achieve a similar therapeutic effect as *patisiran*, the

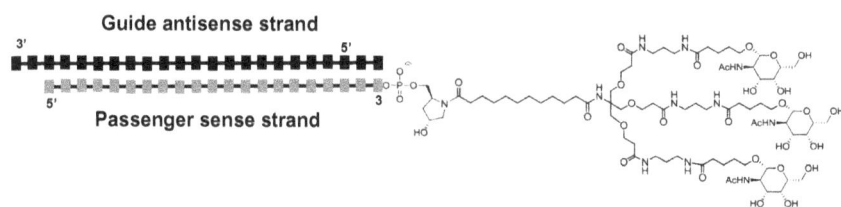

**Figure 11.5.** Structure of *vutrisiran*. The ternary N-acetylgalactosamine (3GalNac) moiety binds to the liver hepatocytes asialoglycoprotein receptor, ensuring siRNA entry into the target cell with high targeting specificity and efficiency.

LNP siRNA developed against the same genetic disease. Polyneuropathy, cardiomyopathy, and wild-type transthyretin amyloidosis are all envisioned as *vutrisiran* indications.

As compared to the LNP formulation used for *patisiran*, GalNac-siRNA conjugate allows simpler GMP preparation and storage conditions, as well as a more convenient administration protocol (SC versus IV). In addition, slow diffusion to capillaries through the extracellular conjunctive tissue creates a "depot" effect, which, together with increased metabolic stability, allows for less frequent administration. Remarkably, the last generation of GalNac siRNAs carrying a phosphate triglycan-end group allows for a treatment regimen as distant as twice a year for multiple indications requiring silencing of a liver-expressed protein. A one-year duration after a single dose has been reported for *cemdisiran*, which holds substantial potential in treating complement-mediated diseases such as paroxysmal nocturnal hemoglobinuria (PNH). This is a historically never-achieved performance. Thus, the GalNac targeting technology actually represents the most promising approach for siRNAs, as illustrated by the fast development of *givosiran* (clinically approved in 2019 for adults with acute hepatic porphyria), *lumasiran* (clinically approved in 2020 for hyperoxaluria type 1), and *nedosiran* (clinically approved in the USA in 2023 for primary hyperoxaluria). Similarly, the GalNac targeting technology is also being pursued for many other applications (Table 11.2) and for delivering ASOs to the liver.

### 11.5.2  *Hypercholesterolemia*

Atherosclerotic cardiovascular disease is the globally leading cause of morbidity and mortality. High-intensity statin therapies, proposed as first-line treatments, are in some cases ineffective or poorly supported, leading to unwanted skeletal muscle side effects. Consequently, a large proportion of patients at risk remains above the LDL-cholesterol (LDL-C) therapeutic threshold, while it is crucial to reduce LDL-C levels for preventing and treating atherosclerotic cardiovascular disease.

The proprotein convertase subtilisin/kexin type 9 (PCSK9) is a protein that regulates the degradation of LDL receptors on the surface of liver cells, thereby affecting LDL clearance from the blood circulation. The PCSK9 protein binds to the LDL receptor and promotes its endocytosis and subsequent lysosomal degradation, thus reducing the number of LDL receptors available for clearing LDL from the blood. This is the rationale for anti-PCSK9 therapy, which has proven to be highly effective in reducing LDL-C levels in humans.

The first clinically approved PCSK9 inhibitors, *evolocumab* (Repatha) and *alirocumab* (Praluent), are both monoclonal antibodies targeting PCSK9. Both medications are used to manage hypercholesterolemia, especially in patients who are unable to achieve their LDL-C goals with statins alone. However, the shortcomings of low compliance and the high cost of monoclonal antibody production remain as the major obstacles to using these drugs for a large number of potentially concerned patients.

*Inclisiran* a promising siRNA therapeutic, targets PCSK9. As for the growing number of therapeutic siRNA, *inclisiran* is based on triGalNac technology mentioned above, which targets hepatocyte asialoglycoprotein receptor (Figure 11.5 and Section 8 of Chapter 6). The *inclisiran* chemical formula is $C_{529}H_{664}F_{12}N_{176}O_{316}P_{43}S_6$, indicating the presence of six phosphorothioate linkages. The formula is further detailed in Table 11.3.

*Evolocumab* and *alirocumab* are administered subcutaneously every two weeks at doses of 140 and 150 mg, respectively, or monthly at doses of 420 and 300 mg, respectively. Strikingly, the chemical modifications introduced in the siRNA *inclisiran* have been so efficient that this treatment requires only two or three injections per year, making it a convenient option for patients in terms of treatment compliance, constant coverage, and, eventually, production cost. *Inclisiran* is administered as a subcutaneous injection given in the abdomen, upper arm, or thigh every 6 months.

**Table 11.3.**   Structural formula of *inclisiran.*

| Sense strand |
| --- |
| 5' _____ 3' |
| Cms-Ums-Am-Gm-Am-Cm-Cf-Um-Gf-Um-dT-Um-Um-Gm-Cm- Um-Um- Um-Um-Gm-Um-L96 |
| **Antisense guide strand** |
| 3' _____ 5' |
| Ams-Ams-Gmu-Am-Um-Cf-Um-Gf-Gm-Af-Cm-Af-Am-Af-Am-Cf-Gm-Af-Af-Af-Ams-Cfs-Am |

The counterion for the negative charges of inter-nucleotide bonds is Na+ in the pharmaceutical preparation. Af = adenine 2'-F ribonucleotide; Cf = cytosine 2'-F ribonucleotide; Gf = guanine 2'-F ribonucleotide; Am = adenine 2'-OMe ribonucleotide; Cm = cytosine 2'-OMe ribonucleotide; Gm = guanine 2'-OMe ribonucleotide; Um = uracil 2'-OMe ribonucleotide; L96 = triantennary GalNAc (N-acetyl-galactosamine). The letter "s" indicates that the following nucleotide is linked through a phosphorothioate bond, two at the 5' end of the sense strand and two at both the 3' and 5' ends of the antisense guide strand.

# 11.6  Allele-Specific Silencing

In gain-of-function dominant-negative disorders, an ideal strategy, for ASO or siRNA-induced mRNA degradation would be to specifically target the variant mutant sequence in the pre-mRNA and mRNA. However, this would require a personalized ASO or siRNA drug for each variant. This might not be feasible for several pharmacological reasons, including the potential toxicity associated with off-target effects of certain specific ASO or siRNA and because of cost considerations. In addition, this strategy is not usable for genetic diseases linked to gene duplication or to triplet repeat expansion such as Huntington's disease (HD; CAG repeat expansion) or spinocerebellar ataxia subtypes (CAG or CTG repeats), in which the available variant sequences that could be targeted are present on both wild-type and mutated genes.

An ASO or siRNA targeting a non-variant sequence on the pathological gene represents the most natural approach for an RNA drug that could ideally treat all patients, independent of their specific variant genotypes.

However, this leads to complete repression of both the wild-type and dominant-negative variant alleles.

The above strategies cannot be applied when at least a minimal expression of the wild-type protein is required. In such a case, allele-specific silencing must be sought. Allele-specific silencing can be achieved by targeting one or several single nucleotide polymorphisms (SNPs) associated with a variant allele in the patient population. This approach is only feasible if common, specific SNPs can be identified in a high percentage of the various mutated alleles within the diseased population. This strategy has been followed in HD and spinocerebellar ataxia.

Epidemiological studies on the HD patient population and targetable SNPs suggest that 80–85% of HD patients could be treated with panels of 2 to 5 SNP heterozygosity, meaning that only the expanded variant allele possesses these 2–5 SNPs in these individuals. Exciting preclinical results obtained with a brain-targeted di-siRNA have been reported with fully chemically modified, therapeutically translatable siRNAs targeting SNP heterozygosity specific to Huntingtin variants. It allowed a 50-fold dis-criminative power for the Huntingtin variant genetic allele in a cell-based assay on human neurons derived from human Huntington chorea patient iPSCs. This optimized siRNA was obtained through repeated, targeted screening and chemical optimization. A selective silencing of the mutant huntingtin HTT allele (>85%) was detected throughout the brain in a HD mouse model using this technology.

Autosomal dominant centronuclear myopathy (AD-CNM, orphanet code ORPHA 169 189) is a rare congenital myopathy characterized by numerous centrally placed nuclei on muscle biopsy. Clinical features are those of congenital myopathy: hypotonia, distal/proximal muscle weak-ness, rib cage deformities sometimes associated with respiratory insuffi-ciency, ptosis, ophthalmoparesis, and weakness of the muscles of facial expression with dysmorphic facial features.

AD-CNM results from heterozygous mutations in the DNM2 gene, which encodes dynamin 2, and to date, 37 mutations (mainly missense) have been identified. Dominant DNM2 mutations also cause rare cases of Charcot–Marie–Tooth (CMT) peripheral neuropathy and hereditary spastic paraplegia. The DNM2 protein belongs to the superfamily of large guanosine triphosphatases (GTPases) and is involved in endocytosis and intracellular vesicle trafficking through its role in the deformation of biological membranes, particularly in muscle cell T-tubule biogenesis. The role of DNM2 as a regulator of actin and microtubule cytoskeletons has also been reported. A potential AD-CNM pathophysiological mechanism is the formation of abnormally stable polymers by mutant Dynamin 2.

A single copy of the wild-type allele in heterozygous knockout mice expressing 50% Dnm2 displays a healthy wild-type phenotype. Moreover, homozygous DNM2 mutation reported in three consanguineous patients leads to a lethal congenital syndrome associated with akinesia, joint contractures, hypotonia, and skeletal abnormalities, together with brain and retinal hemorrhages. These and other data point to the necessity of an allele-specific siRNA drug that silences only the dynamin 2 variant, thereby maintaining 50% of dynamin 2 production.

The proof of concept for silencing the variant mRNA without affecting the wild-type transcript has been obtained in a mouse model using a shRNA gene delivered via an AAV virus. A complete rescue of the muscle phenotype was maintained for at least one year after a single injection of the shRNA AAV, leading to a sustained reduction of the variant *Dnm2* transcript. This study also suggested a new potential pathophysiological mechanism linked to mutant protein accumulation with age, which does not occur in wild-type animals and which can be prevented by shRNA treatment.

Further progress was obtained by screening a library of siRNAs targeting specific heterozygous SNPs associated with the DNM2 dominant-negative variant gene in the AD-CNM patient population. About 75% of patients could be covered by four different siRNAs targeting the four SNPs most frequently associated in a heterozygote manner among the AD-CNM patient population.

One allele-specific siRNA strategy is now in a clinical trial for the treatment of pachyonychia congenita, a rare skin disorder linked to a dominant-negative mutation in keratin 6a. Expanding approaches of allele-specific siRNA technology are being actively developed.

## 11.7 Combined RNA Drug Silencing and Replacement Gene Therapy

For the gain-of-function disorders related to triplet expansions, which have been discussed in the preceding section, an alternative approach has been proposed that does not require the presence of a specific SNP on the heterozygote variant allele. The strategy is based on simultaneous knockdown of both pathologic variant and healthy wild-type endogenous mRNAs, together with the administration of a gene encoding the correct wild-type protein. The replacement gene sequence must be codon-optimized using the genetic code degeneration to accommodate differences with the endogenous human gene, thereby enabling it to be discriminated and untargeted by therapeutic silencing ASO, siRNA, or shRNA. Additionally, codon optimization might also contribute to ensuring a high expression level of the wild-type protein.

Oculopharyngeal muscular dystrophy (OPMD) is a rare muscle disease characterized by an onset of weakness in the pharyngeal and eyelid muscles. Inherited in an autosomal dominant mode, the disease is found on all continents, with several clusters identified in Quebec and Israel. The clinical diagnosis is confirmed by a genetic test, which, in most cases, shows an 11–18 expansion of GCA or GCG triplets in the gene of poly(A) Binding Protein Nuclear 1 (PABPN1) on chromosome 14. The disease is caused by the extension of the polyalanine tract in the PABPN1 protein, leading to the gain-of-function formation of intranuclear inclusions or aggregates in the muscles of OPMD patients, which are the hallmarks of the disease. Although PABPN1 is ubiquitously expressed and contributes to control gene expression in all tissues, playing key roles in mRNA post-transcriptional processing, polyadenylation, RNA decay, and gene regulation, the phenotype linked to PABPN1 pathological variants is restricted to a limited set of skeletal muscles affected in OPMD. The exact pathophysiological process leading to the localized pathology and the precise role of intranuclear aggregates remain unclear.

In a gene therapy approach, two AAV vectors were co-delivered, the first expressing a cassette, including a triple shRNA under the control of an RNA polymerase III promoter, and the second expressing human codon-optimized PABPN1 under the control of a skeletal and cardiac muscle-specific promoter. This treatment significantly reduced the amount of muscle cell nuclei containing PABPN1-positive insoluble intranuclear inclusions, led to significant improvements in several histopathological features (muscle regeneration, fibrosis, and muscle force), and almost completely nomalized muscle cell transcriptome.

Subsequent work managed to condense the two AAV vectors into one and reported reversion of already established insoluble aggregates and partial muscle rescue from atrophy, which are both crucially important since, in most cases, OPMD patients already have an established disease when diagnosed. Also reported were the prevention of muscle fibrosis formation and stabilization of muscle strength to a healthy level. Recent progress toward a clinical trial described a unique single bifunctional construct under the control of a muscle-specific promoter for the co-expression of both the codon-optimized PABPN1 protein and and siRNA against wild-type PABPN1 sequence. A single intramuscular injection of the AAV9 vector in a murine model resulted in the inhibition of mutant PABPN1 and PABPN1 replacement, leading to in vivo restoration of normal levels of muscle strength and other muscle parameters.

# Bibliography

### *About interference*

Boivin M, Charlet-Berguerand N. Trinucleotide CGG repeat diseases: an expanding field of polyglycine proteins? *Front genet*. 2022 Feb 28;13:843014. doi: 10.3389/fgene.2022.843014.

Elbashir SM, Harborth J, Lendeckel W, Yalcin A, Weber K, Tuschl T. Duplexes of 21-nucleotide RNAs mediate RNA interference in cultured mammalian cells. *Nature*. 2001;411:494–8.

Fire A, Xu S, Montgomery MK, Kostas SA, Driver SE, Mello CC. Potent and specific genetic interference by double-stranded RNA in Caenorhabditis elegans. *Nature*. 1998 Feb 19;391(6669):806–11. doi: 10.1038/35888.

Montgomery MK, Xu S, Fire A. RNA as a target of double-stranded RNA-mediated genetic interference in Caenorhabditis elegans. *Proc Natl Acad Sci U S A*. 1998 Dec 22;95(26):15502–7. doi: 10.1073/pnas.95.26.15502.

## *About siRNA*

Brunet de Courssou JB, Durr A, Adams D, Corvol JC, Mariani LL. Antisense therapies in neurological diseases. *Brain*. 2022 Apr 29;145(3):816–31. doi: 10.1093/brain/awab423.

Conroy F, Miller R, Alterman JF, Hassler MR, Echeverria D, Godinho BMDC, Knox EG, Sapp E, *et al*. Chemical engineering of therapeutic siRNAs for allele-specific gene silencing in Huntington's disease models. *Nat commun*. 2022 Oct 3;13(1):5802. doi: 10.1038/s41467-022-33061-x.

Dicerna. Methods and compositions for the specific inhibition of transthyretin (TTR) by double-stranded RNA. *US Pat Trademark Off*. US20190144859, 1–240 (2019).

Dudhal S, Mekzine L, Prudhon B, Soocheta K, Cadot B, Mamchaoui K, Trochet D, Bitoun M. Development of versatile allele-specific siRNAs able to silence all the dominant dynamin 2 mutations. *Mol ther nucleic acids*. 2022 Aug 13;29:733–48. doi: 10.1016/j.omtn.2022.08.016.

Echaniz-Laguna A, Cauquil C, Labeyrie C, Adams D. Treating hereditary trans-thyretin amyloidosis: present & future challenges. *Rev neurol*. 2022 Sep 20:S0035-3787(22)00742-1. doi: 10.1016/j.neurol.2022.07.006.

Elkayam E, Parmar R, Brown CR, Willoughby JL, Theile CS, Manoharan M, Joshua-Tor L. siRNA carrying an (E)-vinylphosphonate moiety at the 5' end of the guide strand augments gene silencing by enhanced binding to human Argonaute-2. *Nucleic acids res*. 2017 May 5;45(8):5008. doi: 10.1093/nar/gkw1298.

Foster DJ, Brown CR, Shaikh S, Trapp C, Schlegel MK, Qian K, Sehgal A, Rajeev KG, *et al*. Advanced siRNA designs further improve in vivo performance of GalNAc-siRNA conjugates. *Mol ther*. 2018 Mar 7;26(3): 708–17. doi: 10.1016/j.ymthe.2017.12.021.

German CA, Shapiro MD. Small interfering RNA therapeutic inclisiran: a new approach to targeting PCSK9. *BioDrugs*. 2020 Feb;34(1):1–9. doi: 10.1007/s40259-019-00399-6.

Gosselin NH, Schuck VJA, Barriere O, Kulmatycki K, Margolskee A, Smith P, He Y. Translational population-pharmacodynamic modeling of a novel long-acting siRNA therapy, inclisiran, for the treatment of hypercholesterolemia. *Clin pharmacol ther*. 2023 Feb;113(2):328–38. doi: 10.1002/cpt.2774.

Holm A, Hansen SN, Klitgaard H, Kauppinen S. Clinical advances of RNA therapeutics for treatment of neurological and neuromuscular diseases. *RNA biol*. 2022;19(1):594–608. doi: 10.1080/15476286.2022.2066334.

Hu B, Weng Y, Xia XH, Liang XJ, Huang Y. Clinical advances of siRNA therapeutics. *J gene med*. 2019 Jul;21(7):e3097. doi: 10.1002/jgm.3097.

Hu B, Zhong L, Weng Y, Peng L, Huang Y, Zhao Y, Liang XJ. Therapeutic siRNA: state of the art. *Signal transduct target ther*. 2020 Jun 19;5(1):101. doi: 10.1038/s41392-020-0207-x.

Kay C, Collins JA, Caron NS, Agostinho LA, Findlay-Black H, Casal L, Sumathipala D, Dissanayake VHW, *et al.* A comprehensive haplotype-targeting strategy for allele-specific HTT suppression in Huntington disease. *Am J Hum Genet*. 2019 Dec 5;105(6):1112–25. doi: 10.1016/j.ajhg.2019.10.011.

Khvorova A, Watts JK. The chemical evolution of oligonucleotide therapies of clinical utility. *Nat biotechnol*. 2017 Mar;35(3):238–48. doi: 10.1038/nbt.3765.

Kosmas CE, Muñoz Estrella A, Sourlas A, Silverio D, Hilario E, Montan PD, Guzman E. Inclisiran: a new promising agent in the management of hypercholesterolemia. *Diseases*. 2018 Jul 13;6(3):63. doi: 10.3390/diseases6030063.

Malerba A, Klein P, Lu-Nguyen N, Cappellari O, Strings-Ufombah V, Harbaran S, Roelvink P, Suhy D, *et al.* Established PABPN1 intranuclear inclusions in OPMD muscle can be efficiently reversed by AAV-mediated knockdown and replacement of mutant expanded PABPN1. *Hum mol genet*. 2019 Oct 1;28(19):3301–8. doi: 10.1093/hmg/ddz167.

Marimani MD, Ely A, Buff MC, Bernhardt S, Engels JW, Scherman D, Escriou V, Arbuthnot P. Inhibition of replication of hepatitis B virus in transgenic mice following administration of hepatotropic lipoplexes containing guanidinopropyl-modified siRNAs. *J Control Release*. 2015 Jul 10;209:198–206. doi: 10.1016/j.jconrel.2015.04.042.

Ranasinghe P, Addison ML, Dear JW, Webb DJ. Small interfering RNA: discovery, pharmacology and clinical development-an introductory review. *Br J Pharmacol*. 2022 Oct 17. doi: 10.1111/bph.15972.

Scherman D, Rousseau A, Bigey P, Escriou V. Genetic pharmacology: progresses in siRNA delivery and therapeutic applications. *Gene ther*. 2017 Mar;24(3):151–6. doi: 10.1038/gt.2017.6.

Schlegel MK, Janas MM, Jiang Y, *et al*. From bench to bedside: improving the clinical safety of GalNAc-siRNA conjugates using seed-pairing destabilization. *Nucleic acids res*. 2022 Jul 8;50(12):6656–70. doi: 10.1093/nar/gkac539.

Springer AD, Dowdy SF. GalNAc-siRNA conjugates: leading the way for delivery of RNAi therapeutics. *Nucleic acid ther*. 2018 Jun;28(3):109–18. doi: 10.1089/nat.2018.0736.

Zhang MM, Bahal R, Rasmussen TP, Manautou JE, Zhong XB. The growth of siRNA-based therapeutics: updated clinical studies. *Biochem pharmacol*. 2021 Jul;189:114432. doi: 10.1016/j.bcp.2021.114432.

Zhang Y, Chen H, Hong L, Wang H, Li B, Zhang M, Li J, Yang L, Liu F. Inclisiran: a new generation of lipid-lowering siRNA therapeutic. *Front pharmacol*. 2023 Oct 13;14:1260921. doi: 10.3389/fphar.2023.1260921.

# Chapter 12

# Challenges and Perspectives of ASOs and siRNA Drugs

## 12.1 Challenges

Synthetic RNA drugs face several challenges and bottlenecks. The first one concerns pharmacodynamic/pharmacokinetic (PK/PD) properties. Except for the liver, delivery of RNA drugs to other organs and tissues is still not performed ideally. Lack of proper delivery of a sufficient amount into the muscles of the *eteplirsen* morpholino ASO might be responsible for its debated performance. Also, CNS delivery of RNA drugs still necessitates intrathecal, intraventricular, or intracerebral administration, which is clinically demanding and associated with infection risk. For muscular and neuromuscular indications, a novel muscle-targeting platform obtained by the conjugation of siRNAs with an anti-CD71 Fab' fragment has been reported. This conjugate led to one-month durable gene silencing in the heart and skeletal muscle after IV administration in normal mice and significant gene silencing when injected intramuscularly. In a mouse model of peripheral artery disease, the IM treatment with an anti-myostatin siRNA resulted in significant silencing of myostatin in muscle, leading to the recovery of the running performance. This technology is now in a clinical trial for a Type 1 myotonic dystrophy RNA drug.

Another PK/PD challenge paradoxically arises from the outstanding efficacy of the last generation of RNA drugs. The remarkable duration of the siRNA silencing effect after a single dose results from its metabolic stability and increased affinity for RISC, which can be attributed to the optimized chemistries described in Chapters 10 and 11. In addition, grafting functional groups, such as 5'vynil phosphonate or methyl phosphonate, facilitates guide strand interaction with the RISC complex. By this method, the guide strand can remain stably bound to RISC and can undergo sustained multiple recycling. The fact that a single administration can lead to 6–12 months of activity raises the necessity to find ways to terminate treatment promptly when required, especially in cases of severe adverse events. Stopping drug effects can be achieved by promoting guide strand dissociation from RISC. Such a reversal system has been described in the liver. It uses short synthetic, high-affinity oligonucleotides complementary to the siRNA guide strand, which can compete with RISC binding to the guide strand. The authors reported that 9-mers with five locked nucleic acids (LNAs) exhibit the highest potency across several targets, enabling them to displace the guide strand from RISC and stop the interference reaction. This 9-mer is targeted to liver hepatocytes through a tri-GalNac moiety.

Attention must also be given to the risk of potential toxicity effects of ASOs/siRNA. The first type of toxicity might result from direct interactions between the ASOs/siRNA and cellular proteins via a hybridization-independent mechanism. This potential toxicity must be characterized in a manner similar to that of any classical drug toxicity.

The hybridization of ASOs, of the siRNA/RISC complex, or of free single-strand siRNA to non-intended RNAs sharing some sequence homology with the target mRNA is called the "off-target effect." For instance, ASO hepatotoxicity in mice has been described to be partly mediated via the RNase H-dependent degradation of off-target RNAs. Some strategies are being developed in order to alleviate the ASO off-target effects. Optimization of the ASO nucleotide length by extending its size from a 14-mer to a 18-mer has been shown to reduce the number of off-target candidates, presumably by decreasing the number of matchings with non-intended mRNAs.

siRNA might suppress the expression of unintended mRNAs with partially complementary sequences through a mechanism similar to that of miRNA-mediated RNA silencing. This siRNA-mediated off-target effect occurs mainly due to similarities in the siRNA seed region (nucleotides 2–8). An in-depth analysis involving a machine learning technique and using a random sampling procedure led to the conclusion that nucleotides 2–5 were mostly responsible for the siRNA off-targert effects on mRNA. Enhanced stabilization chemistry has recently been proposed to substantially reduce siRNA's seed-mediated binding to off-target transcripts while maintaining its on-target activity.

Another cause of off-target silencing is improper strand selection by RISC. Passenger-strand silencing can be avoided by selecting siRNA sequences with high thermodynamic asymmetry or by chemically modifying the sense strand, as described in Chapter 10.

Abundant siRNAs or shRNAs can overload the endogenous RNAi silencing pathway, leading to toxicity, which has mainly been reported in hepatocytes. Precise dosing must be carefully optimized to avoid saturation of the RISC system and limit hepatotoxicity of short- and long-term clinical gene silencing by either approach.

Other challenges for the future of synthetic ASO and siRNA drugs originate from the rapid advance of alternative techniques such as viral gene therapy for delivering an shRNA, which leads to the same effect as ASO and siRNA in terms of steric blockers for exon skipping or translation inhibition and for inducing mRNA cleavage/degradation. Indeed, currently, most proofs of concept for RNA drugs have been obtained at the laboratory scale using specifically designed shRNAs delivered by AAV or lentivirus vectors. However, this gene therapy approach is less flexible than synthetic ASOs and siRNA because no temporal conditional expression system has been clinically approved as yet, which renders hazardous the control of gene therapy treatment termination. Moreover, synthetic compounds might be preferable in terms of production costs. Finally, synthetic RNA drugs can be administered repeatedly without initiating any immune response, whereas distinct viral serotypes must be used for the multiple administration of viral vector doses.

A significant challenge to ASO and siRNA use arises from the fact that genome editing, as a rapidly evolving technology, may advantageously replace mRNA extinction by ASOs or siRNA. Targeted DNA double-strand breaks (DSBs) using CRISPR-Cas9 have revolutionized genetic intervention, enabling efficient and accurate genome editing in a broad range of eukaryotic systems. Multiple applications are actively being investigated, such as targeted knock-out of dominant negative pathological genes or viral genomes, either integrated or episomal (see Chapter 9). Since LNPs can efficiently deliver CRISPR-Cas9 to the liver, many ASO and siRNA indications might eventually also be treated using this genome editing technology. More time is necessary however to assess the safety of this approach in the long term, especially concerning off-target effects, genotoxicity, and germ-line modification, since CRISPR-Cas9 makes cuts in the genomic DNA in contrast to ASOs and siRNA, which target mRNA. Also, genome editing represents an irreversible therapy through a knock-out of the targeted gene. Thus, the pros and cons of genome editing must be weighed for each specific indication in comparison to reversible synthetic RNA drugs.

## 12.2  Perspectives

The examples detailed in Chapters 10 and 11 illustrate the wide and versatile capacities of antisense and siRNA technologies. A large additional number of diseases could potentially benefit from ASO and siRNA drugs. Without being by any means exhaustive, one can mention several other diseases where specific silencing has shown benefits in preclinical models. In facioscapulohumeral muscular dystrophy (FSHD), the knockdown of the FSHD region gene 1 (FRG1) was achieved using miRNAs, delivered using an AAV vector system. The AAV2/9-mediated delivery of a shRNA targeting the Pmp22 mRNA, when injected into the sciatic nerve, prevented the development of pathological features in a rat model of Charcot–Marie–Tooth disease 1A. An allele-specific RNA interference using an AAV9 has been described in a Charcot–Marie–Tooth disease type 2D mouse model. RNAi sequences targeting the dominant mutant of glycyl-tRNA synthetase (GARS) mRNA, but not the wild type, were optimized and then packaged into AAV9 for *in vivo* delivery. This prevented neuropathy in mice treated at birth. However, delaying treatment until after disease onset drastically reduced the benefits of gene therapy, and its therapeutic effects decrease with a delay in treatment, which points to the value of early diagnosis. In most cases, the proof of concept was obtained using shRNA delivered by an AAV vector because this is easily obtained at the laboratory level and because several AAV serotypes display suitable organ penetration and accessibility. An AAV shRNA proof of concept then opens the way to searching for synthetic genetic ASOs or siRNA drugs.

Genetic pharmacology with synthetic ASO or RNA drugs, which is also sometimes considered gene therapy, has shown impressive progress after 20 years of relentless and intensive efforts to improve RNA drug performances. Two to three logs enhancement of their potency has led to recent extraordinary successes, such as being able to silence a pathological gene by a twice- or even once-a-year subcutaneous administration of milligram amount of the compound, which represents an historic performance never reached before by a chemical drug.

The ASO and siRNA drug technology platform, whose chemistry is still continuously improving, is very versatile and can be applied to a large variety of therapeutic applications once the first proof of concept has been obtained, including for decreasing the expression or completely silencing previously non-druggable proteins. Of particular value for rare diseases is the possibility of tackling dominant negative gain-of-function genetic diseases, among which are those linked to triplet expansions. Trinucleotide repeat diseases lead to either toxic RNA or toxic protein products, and they represent a widening class of rare diseases which are not only restricted to the ones illustrated in the preceding chapters, including Type 1 myotonic dystrophy, centronuclear myopathy, Huntington chorea, and spinocerebellar ataxia, but also cover other triplet extension expanding disease families.

The LNP mRNA vaccine technology can be rapidly adapted to any new pathogen by administering pathogen-specific mRNA sequences through a general delivery technology platform and could thus be rapidly applied to mitigate the spread of the COVID-19 pandemic. Similarly, RNA drug improvements have general and extendable perspectives, such as modifications to the phosphodiester linkage, sugars, and nuclei bases. However, it must be stressed that the number and respective positions of the linkages, ribose, and base modifications require a tailor-made optimization, which might be specific for each antisense sequence.

The tri-GalNac targeting has now demonstrated its extraordinary efficacy to deliver RNA drugs to the liver. The majority of present clinical trials concerning RNA drugs benefit from this technology, not only for rare metabolic or neuromuscular disorders such as transthyretin amyloidosis and blood disorders such as hemophilia but also for diseases concerning a much larger portion of the population, such as hypercholesterolemia (by targeting the PCSK9 gene), hypertension, diabetes, and chronic hepatitis.

In parallel to this extension of ASOs and siRNA drug applications to high-prevalence diseases, the technology shows potential to treat an increasing number of severely debilitating or life-threatening ultrarare diseases, which may affect only a handful of patients worldwide. They are referred to as "N-of-1" treatments. The potential of ASO and siRNA drugs to benefit this ultrarare disease population is now raising increasing interest among scientists, GMP drug producers, and regulatory authorities. Since there might be little or no commercial value for these unmet medical needs, patient advocacy groups, charities, and foundations are at the forefront of this challenge.

As a first example, the ASO Milasen was developed to treat a single six-year-old patient with neuronal ceroid lipofuscinosis 7, a neurodegenerative lysosomal storage disorder originating from excessive accumulation of pigment lipofuscin in the body's tissues. Remarkably, the molecular diagnosis of this fatal condition led to the quick, rational design, testing, and manufacturing of the splice-modulating antisense ASO specifically tailored for this unique patient. Proof-of-concept experiments in cell lines from the patient served as the basis for launching the N-of-1 clinical trial of Milasen within one year after first contact with the patient.

More N-of-1 ASO drugs have been developed through accelerated regulatory pathways for specific forms of ataxia-telangiectasia and amyotrophic lateral sclerosis (ALS). It is worth mentioning that gene editing is also making progress toward treating N-of-1 diseases, such as in the case of a rare mutation of Duchenne muscular dystrophy. Treating N-of-1 diseases with personalized therapy — unthinkable a few years ago — is now becoming a reality due to the availability of well-mastered technological platforms which drastically accelerate medicinal development while also reducing costs. This personalized medicine perspective for N-of-1 patients could represent the hallmark of the ongoing genetic drug revolution. However, this will necessitate solving the main obstacle to the generalization of ASO, siRNA, and genome-editing drug use, which consists of identifying efficient delivery methods to all tissues and cell types.

# Bibliography

Alagia A, Eritja R. siRNA and RNAi optimization. *Wiley Interdiscip Rev RNA.* 2016 May;7(3):316–29. doi: 10.1002/wrna.1337.

Boivin M, Charlet-Berguerand N. Trinucleotide CGG repeat diseases: an expanding field of polyglycine proteins? *Front Genet.* 2022 Feb 28;13:843014. doi: 10.3389/fgene.2022.843014.

Bramsen JB, Pakula MM, Hansen TB, Bus C, Langkjær N, Odadzic D, Smicius R, Wengel SL, Chattopadhyaya J, Engels JW, Herdewijn P, Wengel J, Kjems J. A screen of chemical modifications identifies position-specific modification by UNA to most potently reduce siRNA off-target effects. *Nucleic Acids Res.* 2010 Sep;38(17):5761–73. doi: 10.1093/nar/gkq341.

Burel SA, Hart CE, Cauntay P, *et al.* Hepatotoxicity of high affinity gapmer antisense oligonucleotides is mediated by RNase H1 dependent promiscuous reduction of very long pre-mRNA transcripts. *Nucleic Acids Res.* 2016 Mar 18;44(5):2093–109. doi: 10.1093/nar/gkv1210.

Cao W, Lia R, Pei X, *et al.* Antibody-siRNA conjugates (ARC): Emerging siRNA drug formulation. *Med Drug Discov.* 2022 Sep;15:100128.

Crooke ST. Meeting the needs of patients with ultrarare diseases. *Trends Mol Med.* 2022 Feb;28(2):87–96. doi: 10.1016/j.molmed.2021.12.002.

Gillmore JD, Gane E, Taubel J, *et al.* CRISPR-Cas9 *in vivo* gene editing for transthyretin amyloidosis. *N Engl J Med.* 2021 Aug 5;385(6):493–502. doi: 10.1056/NEJMoa2107454.

Glineburg MR, Todd PK, Charlet-Berguerand N, Sellier C. Repeat-associated non-AUG (RAN) translation and other molecular mechanisms in Fragile X Tremor Ataxia Syndrome. *Brain Res*. 2018 Aug 15;1693(Pt A):43–54. doi: 10.1016/j.brainres.2018.02.006.

Kanasty RL, Whitehead KA, Vegas AJ, Anderson DG. Action and reaction: the biological response to siRNA and its delivery vehicles. *Mol Ther*. 2012 Mar;20(3):513–24. doi: 10.1038/mt.2011.294.

Kasuya T, Hori S, Watanabe A, Nakajima M, Gahara Y, Rokushima M, Yanagimoto T, Kugimiya A. Ribonuclease H1-dependent hepatotoxicity caused by locked nucleic acid-modified gapmer antisense oligonucleotides. *Sci Rep*. 2016 Jul 27;6:30377. doi: 10.1038/srep30377.

Kim J, Hu C, Moufawad El Achkar C, Black LE, Douville J, Larson A, Pendergast MK, *et al*. Patient-customized oligonucleotide therapy for a rare genetic disease. *N Engl J Med*. 2019 Oct 24;381(17):1644–52. doi: 10.1056/NEJMoa1813279.

Lombardi MS, Jaspers L, Spronkmans C, *et al*. A majority of Huntington's disease patients may be treatable by individualized allele-specific RNA interference. *Exp Neurol*. 2009 Jun;217(2):312–9. doi: 10.1016/j.expneurol.2009.03.004.

Shen W, De Hoyos CL, Sun H, Vickers TA, Liang XH, Crooke ST. Acute hepatotoxicity of 2' fluoro-modified 5-10-5 gapmer phosphorothioate oligonucleotides in mice correlates with intracellular protein binding and the loss of DBHS proteins. *Nucleic Acids Res*. 2018 Mar 16;46(5):2204–17. doi: 10.1093/nar/gky060.

Treatment of a Single Patient With CRD-TMH-001. https://clinicaltrials.gov/ct2/show/NCT05514249 (last access April 2023).

Yasuhara H, Yoshida T, Sasaki K, *et al*. Reduction of off-target effects of gapmer antisense oligonucleotides by oligonucleotide extension. *Mol Diagn Ther*. 2022 Jan;26(1):117–27. doi: 10.1007/s40291-021-00573-z.

Zlatev I, Castoreno A, Brown CR, Qin J, Waldron S, Schlegel MK, Degaonkar R, Shulga-Morskaya S, *et al*. Reversal of siRNA-mediated gene silencing in vivo. *Nat Biotechnol*. 2018 Jul;36(6):509–11. doi: 10.1038/nbt.4136.

# Supplementary Material

The supplementary material includes:

(a) lecture slides,
(b) quiz.

Online access is automatically assigned if you purchase the ebook online via www.worldscientific.com. If you have purchased the print copy of this book or the ebook via other sales channels, please follow the instructions below to download the files:

1. Register for an account or log in at: www.worldscientific.com/.
2. Go to: https://www.worldscientific.com/r/q0516-supp or scan the QR code below.

3.  Download the files from: https://www.worldscientific.com/worldsci-books/10.1142/q0516#t=suppl.

For subsequent access, simply log in with the same login details in order to access.

For enquiries, please email: sales@wspc.com.sg.

# Index